Curriculum Revolution:
Community Building and Activism

Curriculum Revolution:
Community Building and Activism

National League for Nursing Press • New York

Pub. No. 15-2398

This book was set in Garamond and Baskerville by Publications Development Company. The editor and designer was Rachel Schaperow. Northeastern Press was the printer and binder. The cover was designed by Lillian Welsh.

Printed in the United States of America

Contents

Foreword

THE CREATION OF COMMUNITY IS A POLITICAL ACT

The papers in this volume were written between August and December 1990, a period of intense emotions for the world as Saddam Hussein invaded Kuwait and President Bush and his circle of advisors decided first to commit American troops to defend the surrounding countries and then to extend their stay and send still more troops. When these papers were delivered in early December, a United Nations resolution had set January 15th as a "deadline" for war to begin.

That date itself distressed many people who could not ignore January 15th as the birthday of this country's most recognized apostle for nonviolence, the Reverend Martin Luther King, Jr. The further irony of this date was not lost on those who attended the Seventh National Conference on Nursing Education. The conference was held in Scottsdale, Arizona, despite some strong feelings to join other organizations in boycotting the state because of a recent vote not to recognize King's birthday, the national holiday of January 15th, as a state holiday. These feelings, in turn, were matched by others who felt that Arizona's decision had been misrepresented and so misunderstood, but in any event Arizona's decision should be respected.

The book has been produced during the weeks the war was first waged and then "won" on TV, and the weeks since then in which the President's men made certain choices regarding what the United States ought or ought not do about the hundreds of thousands of refugees fleeing Iraqi retribution.

The book is now published as the United States faces challenges in domestic policy as great as those in foreign affairs. For as surely as the people in the Persian Gulf area need assistance to rebuild their countries, so, too, do the people of the United States where too many live unhealthy lives in unhealthy communities for us to proclaim ourselves a moral and free nation. While the conference planning committee—Gloria Clayton, Nancy Diekelmann, Joyce Murray, Janet Quinn, Sheila Ryan, Christine Tanner, Verle Waters—would have surely chosen a more peaceful context for the discussion of community building, they could not have chosen a more illuminative one for the topic at hand.

INTERNATIONAL COMMUNITY

Could there possibly be a more painful and confusing time than now for the world community, in daily witness to starving, freezing, terrified, yet courageous Kurds seeking refuge? The faces and voices of these people, their children, and their elderly, are forever branded on our collective consciousness and conscience, etching themselves into scars both recent and long formed, scalding away whatever other marks were there that allowed us to recognize ourselves as a humanitarian and just civilization.

Only a few months earlier and several miles to the south of the border the Kurds now seek to cross, a coalition of nations justified a massive military operation on the basis of preserving freedom for the people of Kuwait. But today, any appeals to a similar morality are subordinated to a political and diplomatic defense of the rights of sovereign nations. In trying to make sense of these recent events, we face competing rationales for action—e.g., moral, political, diplomatic—and competing definitions of what constitutes victory and for whom. In addition, if we are strong enough to engage in this painful discussion, we are confronted with competing claims and disclaimers of who is most appropriately responsible for the future of the Kurdish people: Iraq with whom they share a country but whose leader prefers otherwise; the United States with whom they share a common enemy but little else; Turkey with whom they share a common geography; or the Kurds themselves whose call for self-determination has long been ignored by those who divided the Arabian Peninsula into the countries we know now.

The questions are: Where and to whom do the Kurds belong? What way of life for the Kurds is acceptable to the international community? It is increasingly clear that the answers will come not from the Kurds but from those with the political authority of definition. This in itself is a lesson, perhaps not to be endorsed but to be learned, about the nature of communities.

As we attempt to integrate what we feel about the war with what we are coming more and more each day to understand about it, certain questions relevant to our discussions about community building emerge. Where does a community begin and end? Who shall be included and who excluded from a community? What are socially accepted ways for members of a community to act among themselves and toward others? How do we create conditions that nurture and protect the individual, the collective, and the relationship between them?

COMMUNITY AND THE CURRICULUM REVOLUTION

Many have joined the debate about the multiple ways to experience and extend the phenomena that have come to be known as the "curriculum revolution." This year's focus on "community building and activism" was a natural extension of those projects which would join our work as educators with that directed toward advancing a more just and caring society. There have been no final answers presented in these ongoing discussions, not because the participants could not come up with answers as quickly as any others but because the commitment has been to opening up nursing education to the richness of its plurality and diversity.

Certain themes, however, have emerged as characteristic of the curriculum revolution: what Chopoorian (1986) calls the "reconceptualized environment" as context and what Bevis and Watson (1989) call the "educative-caring paradigm" as pedagogy; an embrace of peace and power as shared by Wheeler and Chinn (1989); a feminist attention to society's structures because, in Lorde's words, ". . . the war against dehumanization is ceaseless" (1984, p. 119); internationalism; a respect for the knowledge embedded in practice; a passion for social activism; the inclusion of those not usually included in the tight little circles of power and privilege enjoyed by the educated elite; and a reference list as different from Bloom's and Bennet's as are apples and bananas. The curriculum revolution is not about any one major change; it is about many. It is about the strength that comes from the collaboration of our differences and the collective commitment to celebration. In *Feminism Without Illusion,* Elizabeth Fox-Genovese says that "justice must derive from a collectivity that grounds its deepest principles of individual right in the collectivity's commitment to honor and protect differences" (1991, p. 241). Even stronger is Lorde who reminds us:

> Can any one of us here still afford to believe that efforts to reclaim the future can be private and individual? . . . Revolution is not a one-time event. It is becoming always vigilant for the smallest opportunity to make a genuine change in established outgrown responses, for instance, it is learning to address each other's differences with respect (1984, pp. 140–141).

Such vigilance, such activism, is as necessary for peace in the Middle East as for the building of our communities.

Patricia Moccia, PhD, RN, FAAN
Executive Vice President
Education and Accreditation
National League for Nursing

REFERENCES

Bevis, E. O., & Watson, J. (1989). *Toward a caring curriculum: A new pedagogy for nursing.* New York: National League for Nursing.

Chopoorian, T. (1986). In Moccia, P. (Ed.). *New approaches to theory development.* New York: National League for Nursing.

Fox-Genovese, E. (1991). *Feminism without illusions: A critique of individualism.* Chapel Hill: University of North Carolina Press.

Lorde, A. (1984). *Seiber outsider.* Freedom, CA: The Crossing Press.

Wheeler, C., and Chinn, P. (1989). *Peace and power: A handbook of feminist process* (2nd ed.). New York: National League for Nursing.

Preface

The chapters forming this volume have been selected from presentations offered at the National League for Nursing's Seventh National Conference on Nursing Education. This book is the fourth in the series documenting the reforms in nursing education that are known as the curriculum revolution. The theme of the seventh national conference was "Curriculum Revolution: Community Building and Activism."

The conference was held in Scottsdale, Arizona, the home of Frank Lloyd Wright's Taliesin West. In "A Frank Lloyd Wright Context for Nursing's Curriculum Revolution," Verle Waters compares the building of a nursing curriculum with the building of a physical structure and likens nursing's curriculum revolution to the revolution in architecture promoted by Wright.

The importance of community building in nursing education and nursing practice arises throughout the book. In "Alice in Wonderland: A Metaphor for Professional Nursing Education," Susan Gunby et al. compare students' experiences in nursing education with Alice's adventures in wonderland. "Life as a student of nursing can be very curious; students may experience a loss of identity, self-doubt, uncertainty." The need for building community between students, between teachers, between each other is discussed further in the chapters by Rheba de Tornyay and Nancy Diekelmann.

The importance of story and narrative—talking to each other, disclosing, communicating—is brought to light in chapters such as Marilyn Krysl's "Sometimes a Person Needs a Story More Than Food to Stay Alive" and Nancy Diekelmann's "The Emancipatory Power of the Narrative."

The need for creating community in nursing practice is shown in real-life examples. Beverly McElmurry, Susan Swider, and Kathleen Norr discuss "A Community-Based Primary Health

Care Program for Integration of Research, Practice, and Education." This program, based in the Chicago inner city, strives "to strengthen grass-roots involvement in determining how to improve the health of people in this community." This chapter asks how students will be able to "appreciate the need for change in health care if we do not provide experiential opportunities for them to grapple with the issues."

Julia Tiffany, in "An Interdisciplinary Clinical Practicum: The Demise of a Successful Community Project," offers her experience to other nurse activists. She warns that "birth is not enough. For a vision or dream to survive and thrive requires commitment and structure that transcends individuals." The necessity of community building can be clearly seen in this chapter.

Conference attendees explored new relationships between academic nursing and local, national, and international communities. In her Foreword to this volume, "The Creation of Community Is a Political Act," Patricia Moccia argues the broader implications inherent in community building and activism. Nonceba Lubanga, in "Nursing in South Africa: Black Women Organize," points to the potential power held by nurses and says "nursing education should be relevant to society, serve a purpose, and promote its own interests."

This book calls for nurses to take the responsibility for, as Sister M. Simone Roach says, "creating communities of caring." In Patricia Moccia's words, vigilance and activism are "as necessary for peace in the Middle East as for the building of our communities."

It is our hope that this book will inspire students, educators, and nurses in practice to take the curriculum revolution to each and every community in the nation.

Rachel H. Schaperow
Editor
Division of Communications
National League for Nursing

Contributors

Pamela Chally, PhD, RN
Assistant Professor
Northern Illinois University
DeKalb, Illinois

Rheba de Tornyay, EdD, RN, FAAN
Professor
Department of Community Health Care Systems
Dean Emerita
School of Nursing
University of Washington

Nancy Diekelmann, PhD, RN, FAAN
Helen Denne Schulte Professor
University of Wisconsin—Madison
Madison, Wisconsin

Regina E. Dorman, MSN, RN
Assistant Professor of Nursing
Kennesaw State College
Marietta, Georgia

Kathryn M. Grams, MN, RNC
Assistant Professor of Nursing
West Georgia College
Carrollton, Georgia

Susan S. Gunby, MN, RN
Dean and Assistant Professor of Nursing
Georgia Baptist College of Nursing
Atlanta, Georgia

Margaret M. Kosowski, MSN, RN
Assistant Professor of Nursing
Kennesaw State College
Marietta, Georgia

Marilyn Krysl, MFA
Professor of English
University of Colorado at Boulder
Boulder, Colorado

Nonceba Lubanga, MPH, RN
Health Services Coordinator
Talbot Perkins Children's Services
Associate for Clinical Nursing
Columbia University
New York, New York

Beverly J. McElmurry, EdD, RN, FAAN
Professor, College of Nursing
University of Illinois at Chicago
Chicago, Illinois

Kathleen Norr, PhD
Assistant Professor
College of Nursing
University of Illinois at Chicago
Chicago, Illinois

Betsy S. Pless, MSN, RN
Assistant Professor of Nursing
Medical College of Georgia
School of Nursing
Athens, Georgia

Sr. M. Simone Roach, PhD, RN
St. John's Hospital
Lowell, Massachusetts

Susan M. Swider, PhD, RN
Clinical Assistant Professor
College of Nursing
University of Illinois at Chicago
Chicago, Illinois

Julia C. Tiffany, EdD, RN
Associate Professor
School of Nursing
University of Southern Maine
Portland, Maine

Verle Waters, MA, RN
Dean Emerita
Ohlone College
Fremont, California

1

A Frank Lloyd Wright Context for Nursing's Curriculum Revolution

Verle Waters

In her thoughtful "Reflections on the Curriculum Revolution" in *Journal of Nursing Education* (1990, September), Chris Tanner draws parallels between the curriculum revolution and the natural history of scientific revolutions. To open this conference, held in the city where the late Frank Lloyd Wright's home and workshop, Taliesin West, is located, I wish to draw parallels between the curriculum revolution and the revolution in American architecture he introduced in the early years of this century. The parallels between Frank Lloyd Wright's ideas about constructing houses and many nurse educators' ideas about constructing curricula have interested me for many years. In fact, I gave a speech entitled "The Organic Curriculum" in 1976 at an Associate Degree Council meeting in Washington, DC. In retrospect, I see that the title was wrong for the times. It may have appeared, since I am from California, that I would be talking about granola and alfalfa sprouts, which were big in those days.

Frank Lloyd Wright came to Scottsdale in 1938 and began building Taliesin—he called it his Western Encampment. For the

1

next 20 years, until his death, Taliesin West was his workplace and also a workshop for aspiring architects.

Wright's ideas about the architecture of public and private buildings were certainly revolutionary. He introduced new language and concepts into the field of architecture as he put forth his ideas about the purposes of a building and the relation a building's characteristics have to the quality of life for the inhabitants who live and work within. I find it exciting to think about my craft—designing education structures—in relation to what Wright had to say about his craft—designing living structures.

He, too, had revolution on his mind. His thinking was shaped by a group of men sitting on the verge of the 20th century, even as now we sit on the verge of the 21st, who had a prescience about the course of human events. They suspected that man's inventions would overwhelm him, that man would lose control of his technology. Even as Carolyn Oiler Boyd said at the first curriculum revolution nurse educator conference in 1988, ". . . we stand vulnerably in the wake of a spiraling system of controls on human irregularity made possible by scientific progress. For some of us, the human condition—what it means to exist, to be alive in a world seized by technology—is an appropriate, even important focus for nursing." Wright saw in 1900, in his words, "a great negation" transpiring in America, a desire to be free of the rigid structures associated with European influences. In his mind, this sweeping negation was only the platform upon which to affirm new principles of life and new concepts of architecture (Wright, 1908).

"What is needed most in architecture today," he wrote, "is the very thing that is needed in life—integrity." "In speaking of integrity in architecture," he continued, "I mean much the same thing that you would mean were you speaking of an individual. Integrity is not something to be put on and taken off like a garment. Integrity is a quality within and of the man himself. So it is in a building" (Wright, 1960, p. 293).

So it is also in a curriculum. A curriculum with integrity, like a Frank Lloyd Wright house, is, again using his words, "a natural performance, one integral to site; integral to environment; integral to the life of the inhabitants. A house integral with the nature of materials, wherein glass is used as glass, stone as stone, wood as wood—and all the elements of environment go into and throughout the house. Into this new integrity, once there, those who live in it will take root and grow" (Wright, 1954, p. 15).

Janet Quinn spoke at last year's conference of integrity in relationships between and among faculty and students, and of the healing effects of such relationships. Comparing Quinn's words as she described the teacher, with Wright's words as he described the architect, could make me a believer in channeling. "To be an architect," Wright says, "one must be a man fully human in nature, an awakened man simultaneously aware of his inner being and his outward behavior and relationships." Organic man possesses "an inner centering which releases a wealth of creative energy to the search for processes and forms appropriate to a holistic vision" (Gutheim, 1975, p. 9).

Em Bevis's insistence, at each presentation she has made at these conferences and in the book she co-authored with Jean Watson, *Toward a Caring Curriculum,* that the revolution de-emphasizes curriculum development and emphasizes faculty development reminds me of Frank Lloyd Wright's insistence that the essence of a building is in the space between the structural components rather than in the actual structural components: the walls and the roof. Elaborating his point, he said the spaces between walls and the purposes and people that would inhabit those spaces were of far greater importance to him than the walls themselves (Wright, 1960).

Pat Moccia speaks of the revolution as being about "de-centering the student"—using a phrase she attributes to Bowers. She sees our students, and ourselves, as sociocultural beings embedded in interdependencies, living complicated lives with connections and roots. At the Taliesins, both East and West, Wright decentralized the various functional parts of the buildings in somewhat the same spirit, "Minimizing indoor passageways, he literally forced himself and his people out into the open for direct bodily sensation of the season of the year, the weather of the moment, the time of their lives" (Gutheim, 1975, p. 4).

Wright said, "no house should ever be on a hill. It should be of the hill. Hill and house should live together, each the happier for the other" (Wright, 1960, p. 173). Curriculum revolutionaries say no curriculum should be in the ivory tower. Nursing practice should inform nursing education, each the happier for the other. Wright pioneered the use of an open plan in a house, letting the outside and the inside become more nearly unified. Our revolutionaries, too, all argue that the outside, the practice world, and the inside, the academic world, must become more nearly unified.

David Allen (1990) wants us to swing the pendulum away from the extreme commitment to content. Em Bevis (1989) wants us to revise curricula, not by debating issues of integration, the format of the care plan, which theorist to use, and where to put what content, but by looking outside at the nature and direction of health care. Wright proclaimed a revolution to say "no" to all conventions, habits, and ready-made phrases in the field of architecture; "no" to all esthetic taboos such as proportion, equilibrium, balance, eurythmic, and other trifles. He drew upon nature itself for his design inspiration. Organic architecture simply means a natural architecture. Organic architecture is individual, warm, and friendly. It is realized with natural materials, and contains an air of mystery. Wright emphasized the nobility of the material, and avoided ornament that was not integral. He said of a house that he wanted "the whole structure intimate and wide upon and of the ground itself" (Wright, 1960, p. 45).

Pat Moccia says the goals of the curriculum revolution include establishing nursing education where people live their lives. "We will not teach our students, as we did earlier in our history, only in places where people go to be sick. Nor will we teach them where we have been most recently, where we have retreated to think. But instead, the praxis of the curriculum revolution will expect that we teach and learn with our students in those places where people live: in homes, in their communities, in long-term care facilities, on the streets, in shelters" (1990, pp. 309–310). Thus it is that we take up the fourth nurse educator conference devoted to the cause, "Curriculum Revolution: Community Building and Activism." I close with one last sentence from Frank Lloyd Wright. Where he says "all my architecture," I say "all of our revolutionary programs," and finish the sentence in his words, "are regional in character, traditional in values, and uniquely modern" (1960, p. 185).

REFERENCES

Allen, D. (1990). The curriculum revolution: Radical revisioning of nursing education. *Journal of Nursing Education, 29*(7), 312–16.

Bevis, E. O. (1989). The curriculum consequences: Aftermath of revolution. In *Curriculum Revolution: Reconceptualizing nursing education* (pp. 115–134). New York: National League for Nursing.

Gutheim, F. (Ed.). (1975). *In the Cause of Architecture: Frank Lloyd Wright.* New York: McGraw-Hill.

Moccia, P. (1990). No sire, it's a revolution. *Journal of Nursing Education, 29*(7), 307–311.

Wright, F. L. (1908, March). Organic architecture looks at modern architecture. *Architectural Record.* Republished in *The cause of architecture: Frank Lloyd Wright,* (F. Gutheim, Ed.). New York: McGraw-Hill.

Wright, F. L. (1954). *The Natural House.* New York: Horizon Press.

Wright, F. L. (1960). *Writings and Buildings.* New York: Horizon Press.

2

Creating Community
Among Nurse Educators

Rheba de Tornyay

In preparing my remarks for this seventh annual conference on nursing education, and the fourth one dedicated to the curriculum revolution, I reviewed the excellent papers comprising last year's conference held in Philadelphia. In the introduction, Christine Tanner (1990) says that never before has there been such a powerful climate for change. Daniel Yankelovich, pollster and analyst, echoes this statement. He compared values between 1950 and 1990 and found extraordinary changes in the entire American value system (Geyer, 1990). He points out that we have gone from production to consumption, from future to the immediate, from sacrifice to greed, from public interest to self-interest, from quality to quantity, from long-term to short-term interests.

After a generation of the "me" mentality of American life, we are coming full circle to the realization that the collective "we" has been systematically and tragically ignored in American life in recent years. Taking this idea from the macrocommunity of America to the microcommunity of our college campuses, there is for the first time in many years a real change toward a new definition of

7

common good, of community, and of a sense of the mutual bonds that bind responsible people to their society. We are changing from an "I want" philosophy to a more collective "we should have." These are exciting words and times, and we must capitalize on the welcome return of this societal ethos.

I like the definition of community described in that wonderful book written by Bellah (1985) and his colleagues, *Habits of the Heart.* They point out that although the word "community" often is used loosely by Americans today, it should be used in the sense of describing a group of people who are socially interdependent, who participate together in discussion and decision making, and who share certain practices that both define the community and are nurtured by it. Communities are not formed quickly or easily. If they were, the conference planning committee would not have devoted a major meeting to this topic.

THE CAMPUS COMMUNITY

In a recent document published by the Carnegie Foundation for the Advancement of Teaching, titled *Campus Life in Search of Community,* the president of the Carnegie Foundation, Ernest Boyer (1990), reflects on the four decades of higher education that he has observed first hand. I identified with his contemplations because I've been around that long also. The 50s were an era in which campus growth was the major theme. Students came in droves, and faculty and administrators acted like funds were available for every innovative purpose (and a few not so innovative). Of greater importance to me as a nursing faculty member was the complacency of my students. I had to devise experiences to help them encounter social inequities. They were a placid bunch who lived by the rules and the campus regulations.

Then came the 60s, and I wished I had not been so vigorous in pointing out the problems of society! This was the era in which students gleefully and willfully folded, spindled, and mutilated their enrollment cards to proclaim they were each a person and not a number. The demands for relevance in the curriculum and in courses echoed in the hallways and at the speakers' platforms.

Many positive changes, even some lasting ones, took place in higher education during this time.

Boyer (1990) says that it would be best to forget the 70s because not much happened except that higher education survived. Yet the 70s were important years for nursing education because they represented growth in our graduate programs, and with that growth came the shared value of research to improve our practice. The 70s also divided our nursing community, however, separating faculty into categories that were not healthy— undergraduate and graduate; teaching and research; theory and practice.

The 80s brought more balance to the campuses and to schools of nursing. We began to focus again on the first degree in nursing, the foundation for our profession. The 80s also brought a new concept to our campuses—accountability. Those of us in publicly supported higher education learned that we could not continue to use the old rhetoric to achieve our goals. Legislators demanded that we assume responsibility for our promises and our actions.

In the 90s we have moved from merely talking about responsibility and accountability. Our students are demanding more community on their campuses. They need and want common purpose. They want involvement in the political structure of their campus and school. They are accepting their obligations to the group. They want the rituals that affirm tradition. This decade has been a long time in arriving, and I believe it will be the best yet for higher education. Our own nursing curriculum revolution is a reflection of the new winds blowing in higher education.

The Carnegie Foundation for the Advancement of Teaching (1990) proposes six principles that provide an effective formula for day-to-day decision making on campus and define the kind of community every college and university should strive to be. Because I find it a useful framework, I will use it in this article. These are the six principles of community the report suggests colleges and universities should strive to achieve:

1. An educationally *purposeful* community, where faculty and students share academic goals and work together to strengthen teaching and learning on the campus.

2. An *open* community, where freedom of expression is uncompromisingly protected and where civility is powerfully affirmed.

3. A *just* community, where the sacredness of the person is honored and where diversity is aggressively pursued.

4. A *disciplined* community, where individuals accept their obligations to the group and where well-defined governance procedures guide behavior for the common good.

5. A *caring* community, where the well-being of each member is sensitively supported and where service to others is encouraged.

6. A *celebrative* community, one in which the heritage of the institution is remembered and where rituals affirming both tradition and change are widely shared.

Educationally Purposeful Community

This principle is fundamental to all the others because it describes a faculty and student group which shares academic goals and works together to strengthen teaching and learning on the campus. The central mission of the academy of higher learning is the generation and transmission of knowledge. How we view community on a campus is, therefore, somewhat different from how we think about community in settings such as a neighborhood, workplace, or civil society (Palmer, 1987). Community on our campuses must be focused on our educational agenda.

In an article in *Change,* Palmer (1987) relates the idea of community to questions about the very nature of knowledge. He asks the central questions we all must ponder as we engage in our mission of knowing, teaching, and learning. How do we know? How do we learn? Under what circumstances do we know and learn? It is his thesis that the very way in which we have traditionally accepted what was *the* manner of knowing is outmoded.

As we all know, the mode of knowing that has dominated higher education is what Palmer calls objectivism. We have learned, through our years of education, to hold knowledge at arm's length. The goal has been to keep the knower from the contamination of subjective biases. This serves to divorce the part of the world known as knowledge from personal life. It is a life "out there" somewhere.

The second characteristic of objectivism is analysis. To know something, one must chop it up into pieces and study each piece, usually separately. Only by dissecting knowledge can it be analyzed and understood.

The third component of objectivism is experimental. We move the pieces about, we see what would happen if we reshaped whatever it is we are studying. This process frequently fragments what we really want to know.

Objective, analytic, experimental; these were the words that described my graduate education at Stanford University School of Education three decades ago. I was steeped in the experimental method, and I believe it safe to say the reports of nursing research of the time also tried hard to use the objective, analytic, and experimental model. If we wanted to be a *real* science, then this was what we had to do. Never mind that most of our significant questions did not lend themselves to these methods. We tried to find a question that would be amenable to a methodology that was respectable.

I want to be clear at this point that I do not believe there is anything inherently wrong with being objective or analytical or with being experimental. Yet, Palmer (1987) argues that when students believe that they can take pieces of the world and carve out a niche for themselves, they begin to report on a world that is not the one in which they, themselves, live. Since nursing's central focus is on how people relate to their environment, Palmer's thesis is an important one for us. This focus brings me to the view of community within the concept of ways of knowing.

Teaching and learning in higher education, as with all education, focus on the individual. The individual is the primary agent of knowing. Yet, knowing and learning are communal acts. They require many brains, many ears and eyes, many experiences. The community of scholars we refer to in higher education requires a continual cycle of discussion. Productive discussions force the participants to listen to divergent views, to argue salient points, to find common grounds that can lead to consensus. Community is a capacity for relatedness, both among persons and with the world of ideas (Palmer, 1987).

The price paid for continuing to focus on individuals in education instead of the community of scholars is competition. Were we to draw a sociogram of the traditional classroom, it would go from student to teacher; from teacher to student. This notion of checking and correcting within the classroom promotes fear and competition.

It is in the seminar where students have direct access to their professors in a setting where dialogues thrive and relationships grow, not just between teachers and students, but among the students themselves. In the classroom students should be encouraged to cooperate, not compete. Group assignments and small group discussions within larger lecture sections underscore the point that cooperation in the classroom is essential. Beyond the classroom, the bringing together of faculty and students in intellectual and social events fosters a common intellectual purpose on campus.

Still, the seminar is not a magic place where cooperation flourishes without nourishment. A hospitable environment for students and faculty alike uses every remark, even if mistaken or seemingly stupid, to build the group and also its contributors. When students begin to accept the fact that every attempt at truth is a major contribution to the larger search for consensual truth, they become empowered to say what they want to say, to expose their ignorance, and to unmask themselves for the greater goal. Teachers, as group facilitators who are comfortable admitting they do not know, sharing feelings, and thinking aloud to show the way one gropes for connections, model the ways in which one seeks truth.

Several years ago I had two experiences that caused me to pause and think of how we foster competition among our students. The first experience was an offer from one of our local hospitals to provide a monetary reward for the graduate student whose research at that institution had most influenced nursing practice. Then being a dean, I never turned down an offer for any money as long as it met the criteria of being moral and legal. I did what we always do: appoint a committee composed of students and faculty. To my astonishment, the committee came back saying that the students did not want to choose a single student, but wanted to celebrate everyone's research. On the basis of their report, the hospital administrator was persuaded to sponsor a research day, followed by a reception paid for with the money allocated for the award. This event started me thinking in a new way.

Soon after that episode came graduation time. For many years we had awarded a certificate and a small check to the student who excelled in either scholarship, or humaneness, or had contributed the most to the student organization. We had separate awards for undergraduates, the RN completion undergraduates, and the graduate programs. The RN completion graduates absolutely refused to single out one student for an award. They, too, felt that it would destroy their colleagial relationships, and they, too, wanted to use the money to celebrate their collective achievement. I began to understand and suspect that women didn't like or want to support competitive events.

The newly emerging epistemologies are promoting promising changes toward the quest for knowledge. Foremost among them is feminist thought, which is primarily about another way of seeing and, therefore, of being in the world (Palmer, 1987). Last year, in her discussion about student-teacher relationships, Symonds (1990) identified the feminist process as allowing for open discourse. She described the approach as one that broke down the traditional dualistic roles in teaching and learning. Through her examples she shared what she described as an exhilarating sense of community and empowerment for all participants that transformed teaching and learning into a process instead of a product.

Although the words are hardly new in educational thought and literature, I can well remember when such "soft" words as intuitive, interactive, relatedness, and feelings were relegated to that class of objectives called affective domain. Even the behaviorists acknowledged their importance, but hastily dismissed them as impossible to measure, and, therefore, being of lesser value than the cognitive descriptors of knowledge. As Mager (1962) says in his best-selling book on preparing instructional objectives:

> This book is not concerned with which objectives are desirable or good. It concerns itself only with the form of a usefully stated objective, rather than with its selection. [pp. xi]

In all fairness, I must say the real purpose for his small book on preparing instructional objectives was to help a programmer specify and communicate those educational intents selected.

Although it is in the classroom where community begins, learning also reaches out to dimensions other than the curriculum (Carnegie Foundation, 1990). In teaching and research the university must forge a closer relationship with the world beyond the campus (Lynton & Elman, 1987). Critics of professional education have seen both undergraduate and graduate programs as having curricula that are too narrowly confined to technical skills, with too much of a gap between theory and practice, too much emphasis on purely cognitive and analytical material, too much abstract classroom work, and too little hands-on experience.

Over 20 years ago Jencks and Riesman (1968) found a low correlation between course grades and occupational success. They described how the affiliation of professional schools with universities has tended to de-emphasize the school's occupational commitments and encourage "a more academic and less practical view of what it is that students" need to know (p. 252). In nursing, we have heard that indictment from our practice communities.

The new demands on the practitioner require educational changes that go beyond a mere reshuffling of the curriculum. Broadening programs by including more pertinent liberal arts subjects and adding problem-centered, multidisciplinary courses is necessary, but is not sufficient. We must help students develop the kind of judgment required for good practice and the ability to consider higher-order implications to deal with the resulting complexity and ambiguity. This calls for a rethinking and revision of the basic approach to career-oriented education. Despite wide use of clinical and other practical components, the primary emphasis today continues to be on content rather than on process, on the acquisition of a body of knowledge rather than on the ability to use it. That emphasis must change (Jencks & Riesman, 1968).

For many years the educational approach reflected the traditional view of professional practice as the systematic application of a set of standardized concepts and analytical methods to a recurrent problem to arrive at a unique solution (Moore, 1970). This positivist view has been the hallmark of the professions. During the past decades nursing, along with more and more occupations, has been striving to achieve professional status by adopting this approach. Knowledge is viewed as hierarchical, and there is a corresponding progression of activities. Commonly known as the "leveling" of knowledge, Schein and Kommers (1972) identify three major components:

1. An underlying basic science or discipline component that provides the fundamental principles of the practice,
2. An applied science component that furnishes the problem-solving procedures, and
3. A skills component that consists of acquiring the ability to utilize the basic and applied knowledge in actual practice.

The major tenet of this approach is that learning precedes doing and that practice is the application of theory. Nursing curricula have been built by including first what is viewed as the pertinent basic sciences, followed by the applied science and technology courses. The curriculum ends with intensive clinical experiences designed to provide opportunities to develop the skills of application. Ever since the end of the apprentice type of education prevalent in nursing education for many years, this dogma has permeated the curriculum and has been required by accreditation standards at all levels. The argument that applied science rests on the foundation of basic science has gone unchallenged, as has the assumption in research endeavors that the more basic and general the knowledge, the higher the status of its producer (Schon, 1983).

Successful practitioners learn while doing. They engage in what Schon (1983) calls "reflection in action" as they interact with their client or with the situation they are facing. During this time they continuously reflect on their activity and adjust each successive step on the basis of this reflection. It is an ongoing feedback process of successive approximation, and an exercise in artistry.

This view of professional activity suggests the need for a substantial change in education. A more applied orientation in the curriculum requires greater use of community practitioners on a part- or full-time basis. It gives support to the wide use of clinical faculty to enrich the teaching of students, and of equal importance, to enhance the ability of academically oriented professors to engage in various clinical activities. Many schools use part-time clinical appointments, but the idea of trade-offs to allow for full-time faculty appointment for clinicians has much merit.

Role of the University in practitioner education. Academic institutions have an obligation to link theory with practice. They would not consider providing practice without relating it to a theoretical framework. In the professional development of nurses in practice, it is imperative that they absorb new theories, new paradigms, and new concepts to understand and apply new techniques. This imperative requires courses and seminars that universities are well qualified to provide. Universities must change the tradition of teaching theoretical ideas abstractly and in isolation from their practical application which practitioners want and need.

Colleges and universities must become considerably more flexible and energetic in responding to the external demands of the communities they serve. The business and private sector expects and wants rapid delivery. Corporate clients will not wait patiently for the lengthy process to which academics have become accustomed and fostered. New academic programs characteristically take months to initiate. A continuing education unit can move much more quickly, but later when the students want and expect academic credit the faculty may be faced with a dilemma. There is a need for a rapid and flexible admission procedure for distant learning sites and other innovative approaches to education.

Faculty involvement in inservice education intensifies new pedagogical demands. When health agencies are asked why they don't use the faculty at their local college for inservice programs, the answer too often is that their nurses are treated as teenage college students. Faculty must be able to relate theory and practice and have a broad perspective on their field of specialization, or the courses they provide will not meet the needs of inservice education. It is necessary for faculty to teach more inductively, to help students generalize from the specific, and to provide intellectual guidance to much more active and demanding learners. To quote Lynton & Elman (1987):

> The expanding university places new demands on faculty. The knowledge needs of modern society require that university faculty become more involved in broader areas of scholarship, in the aggregation, synthesis, interpretation, and application of knowledge, and in outreach and extension. In short, faculty must be in contact with the world outside academia. This is also needed to respond to the new lifelong educational needs of employees and professionals. Thus we find again, as in traditional universities, a fundamental relationship between the scholarly activities of faculty and their teaching. It used to be that research, narrowly defined, was seen as important to effective teaching within the confines of the discipline. Now we recognize that scholarly activity in the broader sense is essential to the larger perspectives and experiences that must inform and illuminate teaching in the modern university. [pp. 109]

Service or Scholarship? In our community of scholars, how do we differentiate between service and scholarship? American universities have a long tradition of requiring the triad of teaching, scholarship, and community service. Of the three, we know that scholarship is the one scrutinized most diligently for promotion and tenure. Lynton and Elman (1987) establish the point that service is a term that has the inescapable overtone of "good citizenship," implying the ability to be engaged for the good of the institution and the community. This is the term that is appropriate for serving on the university's library board, or the faculty club board, or on other committees. It is interesting that when we talk about promoting the sense of community, of the triad of faculty expectation this is the one that usually gets the shortest shrift from faculty and administrative review committees. We must be careful not to use the same label for professionally based technical assistance and policy analysis for a local government or community group because these activities are direct applications of the faculty member's professional and scholarly expertise. By contrast, civic involvement, on or off campus, engages the faculty member as a participant within a community and is usually not explicitly based on her or his professional capacity. These are important distinctions in differentiating what faculty members should do as scholars and professionals, on the one hand, and what they should do in their capacity as citizens of the institution and community on the other.

Professional activity is an extension of traditional scholarship. The reward for faculty engaged in such activity does not imply a reduction in the importance of traditional scholarship. Instead, traditional scholarship is enhanced through externally oriented professional activities. It is also important to stress that no one faculty member can be expected to be engaged in the full spectrum of scholarly activities, although the school of nursing faculty as a corporate body must be involved in the full range of activities. Applied professional activities must receive equity in the reward structure. Developing criteria and exemplars for excellence in these activities is the responsibility of each faculty in each school.

One of my academic idols is Donald Kennedy, the president of Stanford University. This institution has greatly influenced my teaching and learning philosophy. Last September, writing for the Stanford community and its alumni, he stated that learning and thinking are the two capacities that must be fused, resonated, and reinforced (Kennedy, 1990). This is the process, he said, through which professors stop being merely teachers and become mentors, and students enter the subtle transition from pupil to apprentice and from apprentice to professional.

The purposeful community of the college or university is fundamental to the academy and to its faculty, students, and staff. Our major purpose is to develop and transmit knowledge. We have undervalued the importance of conveying knowledge and of generating a new generation of scholars through the powerful and demanding task of teaching. The importance of gaining prestige for good teaching on our campuses was the subject of an article in *The Chronicle of Higher Education* (Watkins, 1990). It was suggested that pedagogy be a subject for scholarly debate on the content of the disciplines.

An Open Community

An open community is one in which freedom of expression is uncompromisingly protected and mannerly, decent behavior is powerfully affirmed (Carnegie Foundation, 1990). Standards of communication must go beyond correct grammar or syntax, even beyond the civility of the message being sent. Communication is a sacred trust. The goal of human discourse must be to both speak and listen with great care and to seek understanding at the deepest level. As our campuses become increasingly diverse, this principle cannot be overstated.

Because of their cultural isolation, many students bring prejudices that serve to filter out the feelings of people from racial, ethnic, and religious backgrounds that differ from their own. In an open community, freedom of expression must be defended, but language that hurts others must be denounced. Good communication includes listening as well as speaking. Respecting the rights and dignity of everyone else must not only be expected, but demanded of students, faculty, and staff.

The social and cultural conditions in which one lives and works influence or determine the quality of academic life. All that surrounds the process of education as it occurs in our colleges and universities affects behavior within the academic community. The spirit of inquiry applied to teaching recognizes teaching as a phenomenon in its own right, not only as a skill included in the knowledge of content. The academic community should have the sense of being joined together in the quest to discover more about effective learning and the teaching that can foster that learning. To achieve this goal, questions about teaching should be encouraged, valued, and deliberated. This is consistent with the spirit of inquiry that should permeate the university's environment and value system. Extending that sense of questioning to instructional issues is basic to the mission of the institution. Scholarship must be perceived as broader than research, with the study and inquiry necessary to effective instruction included, particularly in the criteria for promotion and tenure.

A Just Community

The community of higher learning is built from the rich resources of its members. It celebrates diversity and seeks to serve the full range of citizens in our society effectively. To do so it must commit to being a just community where the sacredness of the person is honored and where diversity is aggressively pursued (Carnegie Foundation, 1990).

What does this mean? A brief historical perspective is in order. Colleges used to be, with few exceptions, designed for the privileged of our society. They catered to the most advantaged, and these advantaged later assumed the positions of power and authority in society. Whereas this statement does not reflect nursing's student population, we know that nursing students are predominantly white. By the turn of the century, however, one out of three Americans will be persons of color. The makeup of the American work force is also changing rapidly. People of color and new immigrants will make up more than 83 percent of the new additions to the work force between now and the year 2000. The increased racial, ethnic, and cultural diversity sometimes leads to conflict and polarization. Sadly, racial tensions are increasing on our campuses, not decreasing.

Successful minority enrollment must be more than access to education. It requires support for students once they are enrolled. This support must be financial and emotional.

A just community is one in which diversity is aggressively pursued. This diversity encompasses class, race, and sexual preferences. Our students face many human and social problems that require vision, compassion, and commitment. These attributes are developed through being a part of a community in which people learn to respect and value one another for their differences, while also defining the values shared by all those who join the university as scholars and as citizens.

A Disciplined Community

A disciplined community helps individuals accept their obligations to the group and is one in which well-defined governance
procedures guide behavior for the common good. A community of
learning is guided by standards of student conduct that define
acceptable behavior and integrate the academic and nonacademic
dimensions of campus life. We have an interesting dichotomy today. Students are given detailed requirements for academic matters. They know what they need to do practically every minute of
their time in classes and courses. They know when, how long, and
what the expectations are for term papers and other independent
assignments. Yet, out of class there is only limited discipline. Once
colleges were highly paternalistic; today, it is hands off the students except during their class time.

The Carnegie Foundation study (1990) recommends that a
college or university be a disciplined community, where there are
appropriate rules governing campus life, and where individuals
acknowledge their obligations to the group. An honor code for
both the scholarly and the civic dimensions of campus life is encouraged. Such codes convey a powerful message about how hon-
esty and integrity form the foundation of a community of learning.

We probably would all agree that self-discipline is an important goal in our educational programs. Health professionals value
discipline. It keeps us on the job when we are tired, when we
don't feel well, when we are discouraged. Empowering students
to make crucial decisions about themselves is an essential part of
self-discipline.

The competitive environment of academia has caused dread-
ful symptoms indicating serious pathology. Examples of cheating,
including falsifying research results, blatant plagiarism, lying, and
other unethical behaviors, are unfortunately not rare. Rather than
brand the instigator of the seedy conduct, although such conduct
certainly should not be condoned under any circumstances, let us
pause a moment to reflect upon the reasons for it. The requirement to produce documented evidence of scholarly activities
has pressured some to meet their goals through questionable and

unethical manners. Who knows what the first step is down that slippery slope? What support can a junior faculty member expect from senior faculty that could prevent an error of judgment that could easily cost a career? A community that places high and sometimes unattainable expectations on its members may find that the weaker members succumb to deviant conduct.

A Caring Community

A caring community is one in which the well-being of each member is sensitively supported and service to others is encouraged. Students, particularly undergraduates, need to feel that they belong. A student put it this way: "We don't want the university to be involved *in* our lives, but we do want them to be concerned *about* our lives" (Carnegie Foundation, 1990).

In many institutions today, students fail to feel connected. The modern campus does not have the intimacy of the family. As students are older and living more self-directed lives, their needs also change. Unfortunately, students are still made to feel like numbers. I am appalled at the number of my undergraduate students who routinely give me their student number when they sign off on their written exercises.

The important factor is how students think and feel about their campus. Do they feel supported? When other social bonds are tenuous, students should discover the reality of their dependence on each other. They need to understand what it means to share and to enjoy the benefits of giving. Community must be built. A caring community enables students to gain knowledge and helps them channel that knowledge to humane ends.

There are other important characteristics of the learning environment within the academic community. Students learn better in a climate of confidence (Moore, 1976). The creation of a positive learning environment occurs when students are given many opportunities to succeed, when their progress is measured regularly in small steps, and when they are motivated to keep trying by the belief of the teacher in their commitment and ability to succeed. Faculty, also, must be given opportunities to succeed and be rewarded for their commitment and determination. They need encouragement from one another and from their department chairpersons and deans.

A positive academic environment rewards diversity. Such an environment recognizes and values instructional alternatives to promote and credit students for their past experiences. A spirit of adventure, of exploration, of discovery, and of the conquest of difficult knowledge and tough decisions permeates the rich atmosphere of this academic setting.

To promote a caring climate of inquiry about teaching, questions should be encouraged and raised routinely and regularly during formal department and committee meetings and should be raised informally among colleagues. The academic schedule needs a time for sharing successes and ideas that sounded good but didn't work in teaching. Circulating ideas about teaching is helpful. Materials are shared not because the faculty needs the help, but because the ideas are informative and interesting. We must build this culture into our programs as we have built in the idea of disseminating research reports. We clip out items or send references to our colleagues whom we know are engaged in a particular research endeavor. We must broaden this practice to include educational impressions, techniques, views, and exciting new ideas. I was intrigued with a statement made in an article in *The Chronicle of Higher Education* (Watkins, 1990) that a professor would never send a grant proposal to a funding agency without asking several colleagues for their opinions, but many faculty members do not think of sharing the syllabus of a new course with their colleagues.

Academic leaders (and this must include faculty on promotion committees and chairpersons and deans) should adopt the principle of saying less and doing more about the importance of teaching. Actions speak more eloquently than words, especially when it comes to rewarding and recognizing teaching. Publications about teaching need to count at promotion and tenure time. After all, teaching and learning are the central mission of any educational institution. Departmental travel funds should be available to faculty interested in attending national meetings on teaching and learning.

Although the motive to evaluate teaching by both students and peers as part of promotion and tenure is commendable and needed, it is important to keep in mind that an excessively evaluative environment inhibits the needed exchange of ideas and information about teaching. An atmosphere of "playing it safe" is to be avoided, as is a competitive climate in which faculty are rivals for scarce permanent positions.

The quest for good teaching is never-ending. Novice teachers cannot be sent to achieve it without help. Skilled chairpersons know this and provide opportunities for mentoring within their departments, bring outside consultants to their institutions, and provide funds for their faculty to travel to meetings and other institutions. It is money well invested.

Our discussion about helping our students to transform the system of healthcare delivery evokes the question of where they will get the needed skills. The skills I am talking about are political skills, the talents needed to help make things happen. This is a complex bag of tricks, one that most of us learned through trial and error. This process can be learned in a more efficient manner with feedback techniques; open, honest, and caring evaluation; and through sharing our own experiences as experts in this process of negotiation and compromise.

The comments made by the students in last year's conference, particularly those published in Danner's (1990) chapter of *Curriculum Revolution: Reconceptualizing the Student-Teacher Relationship,* were revealing. Can a caring environment exist where the rules are broken without regard for the recipient? Negative examples exist on every campus: courses cancelled, schedules changed, locations changed, instructors switched. No, these may not be earthshaking problems when one is a faculty member, but don't you remember when you had to figure out how you could work, manage your family, maintain your health, and at the same time be a student?

A contract is an agreement between two parties. When students come to the campus community they have every right to believe that they will receive the education they expect. They have every right to believe that the written contract, in terms of school bulletins and other written materials, is accurate and will be adhered to. The further one goes in education, the more faculty appear to promote the blueprint of an independent program for each student. Designing their own programs helps students develop the negotiation skills I spoke about previously.

We spend considerable time in nursing education promoting the idea of autonomy, or self-determination, for our clients. Students are not always on the receiving end of this important ethical principle. I have been using contract grading for the past five years and wish I had been flexible enough in my younger days to have adopted it sooner. Giving my students the power to decide their grades takes me out of the role of holding the rewards and punishments. It fosters a collegial relationship in the classroom, and allows me freedom to be the facilitator of learning instead of the evaluator.

A Celebrative Community

In a celebrative community we share and remember the heritage of the institution through celebrations and rituals affirming both tradition and change. Colleges need to sustain a keen sense of their heritage and traditions. Nursing on our college campuses is somewhat young. Nursing went through a time when its older traditions were shunned, and the sense of community suffered. I remember when pinning as a completion symbol was abandoned as not being "collegiate" enough.

We must use the knowledge gained from the study of anthropology. The celebrative community uses commemoration and ritual to recall the past, to affirm tradition, and to build larger loyalties. I love the pageantry of campus commencements. They may be from the middle ages, but they give a sense of history and accomplishment to our students and parade them before their parents, spouses, children, and friends in a proud and collective ceremony. The separate nursing completion ceremony, particularly for those students completing their initial professional degree, but to some extent for all students, is a rite of passage that serves to mark the initiation into the profession or a graduation to a new vista. I also favor nursing oaths that bind us to the ethical beliefs and values of our profession in an open and public arena.

Celebrations should occur often during the year. When we celebrate scholarship we confirm it, we make it public, and we show our appreciation to those members of the community who achieve the values we cherish. When we celebrate clinical excellence we again affirm our belief in its importance and publicly honor its recipients.

I can remember when the only celebrations that took place among nursing faculty were those surrounding vital events— mainly marriages and babies. I have nothing against either, but those are personal events. Celebrating a successful research proposal, an even greater event such as getting funded for a successful proposal, a publication, a major appointment—these are activities that should be esteemed, acclaimed, and renowned. One colleague's success reflects on all in the community. My department begins each meeting with a variation on "let's share" and we use all opportunities to celebrate each other in warmth and colleagueship.

CONCLUSIONS

All the factors I've discussed in this paper are interrelated. We have talked endlessly about empowering nurses to be social activists, but we have not empowered our students to help make needed changes in their education. The final speaker last year, Venner Farley (1989) said that we desperately need to change power relationships to help develop the self-esteem so essential for being a professional. Community building is characterized by cooperation among the members. Nursing schools can show the way for the rest of the academy by enhancing the new paradigm of being a community of scholars. We must stop conforming to the traditional ways of knowing, and promote our feminist philosophy and our caring mission. Nursing faculty and students must bring their expertise to their universities and colleges to create a new ideal.

There is no better place to learn political activism than in the academic senate of our respective institutions. Woodrow Wilson once said that he didn't learn the ways of politics in Washington, but from his role as a professor at Princeton. Instead of complaining that some of our values are not internalized by our organizations, we must see that the answer lies in changing our institutions. Like the old advertisement for Purex, academia needs the woman's touch. Who better to give it than nursing faculty?

REFERENCES

Bellah, R. N., Madsen, R., Sullivan, W. M., Swidler, A., & Tipton, S. M. (1985). *Habits of the heart*. New York: Harper & Row.

Boyer, E. L. (1990). Foreword. In Carnegie Foundation for the Advancement of Teaching, *Campus life in search of community* (pp. xi–xiii). Princeton, NJ: Carnegie Foundation.

Carnegie Foundation for the Advancement of Teaching. (1990). *Campus life in search of community*. Princeton, NJ: Carnegie Foundation.

Danner, K. C. (1990). Our voices, our visions. In *Curriculum revolution: Redefining the student-teacher relationship* (pp. 37–45). New York: National League for Nursing.

Farley, V. M. (1990). Clinical teaching: A shared adventure. In *Curriculum revolution: Redefining the student-teacher relationship* (pp. 87–93). New York: National League for Nursing.

Geyer, A. G. (1990, August 2). The concept of community may be making a comeback. *Seattle Times*, pp. A–8.

Jencks, C., & Riesman, D. (1968). *The academic revolution*. Chicago: University of Chicago Press.

Kennedy, D. (1990). Learning, thinking, believing. *Stanford, 18*(3), 27–29.

Lynton, E. A., & Elman, S. E. (1987). *New priorities for the university*. San Francisco: Jossey-Bass.

Mager, R. F. (1962). *Preparing instructional objectives*. Palo Alto, CA: Fearon.

Moore, W. (1970). *The professions*. New York: Russell Sage Foundation.

Moore, W. (1976). Increasing learning among development education students. In J. B. Hefferlin & O. Lenning (Eds.), *Improving educational outcomes: New directions for higher education (#16)*. San Francisco: Jossey–Bass.

Palmer, P. J. (1987). Community, conflict, and ways of knowing. *Change, 19*(3), 20–25.

Schein, E. H., & Kommers, D. W. (1972). *Professional education*. New York: McGraw-Hill.

Schon, D. A. (1983). *The reflective practitioner*. New York: Basic Books.

Symonds, J. M. (1990). Revolutionizing the student-teacher relationship. In *Curriculum revolution: Redefining the student-teacher relationship* (pp. 47–55). New York: National League for Nursing.

Tanner, C. A. (1990). Introduction. In *Curriculum revolution: Redefining the student-teacher relationship* (pp. 1–4). New York: National League for Nursing.

Watkins, B. T. (1990, October 31). To enhance prestige of teaching, faculty members urged to make pedagogy focus of scholarly debate. *The Chronicle of Higher Education, 27*(9), A11–12.

3

Sometimes a Person Needs a Story More Than Food to Stay Alive

Marilyn Krysl

Let me begin with a story.

> I was standing in the corridor outside a patient's room. I knew she would be dead soon. The blind was down. It was so damn dark. I looked at my watch. It was four fifteen, a mid-January four fifteen. Suddenly I saw a line of light—the sun peeking in from the side of the window, sneaking along the floor, climbing up the side of the bed, falling into the patient's hand. I stood there gazing; I was in a dream. Then I heard the patient move a little. I looked are her. She was looking at the light on her hand. She was moving her hand into the light, out of it. She was smiling a little, playing with light, before the darkness took her. [Coles, 1989, p. 101]

This story, which might easily have been told by a nurse, was told to social anthropologist Coles by a busy resident. The resident was grateful for this story and eager to pass it on. He had committed himself to a stressful profession, one in which it would not be easy for him to take good care of himself. He understood he would need many more stories like this one in order to do his work and at the same time to stay human, to stay alive. As nature writer Lopez (1990) says in his book *Crow and Weasel,* "The stories people tell have a way of taking care of them. . . . Sometimes a person needs a story more than food to stay alive."

What is it about stories that is healing? Why is a story more satisfactory than the truth presented in statistics? What does a story give us that a newspaper article or the evening news does not?

Here, for instance, is a piece of data. "Although Caucasian women in the United States abuse drugs in higher proportion and more frequently than do women of color, women of color are ten times more likely than white women to be reported for drug abuse." This is an important piece of data certainly, and we can reason from it that racial discrimination exists and that there is injustice in the world. But this piece of data cannot help us. It cannot help us because it speaks only to a tiny part of us, our intellect and the most minimal range of our emotions. There is no life in this piece of data. We do not ourselves encounter these women, hear their voices, learn their stories. By this piece of data we cannot know them. Life is eliminated from data in order to give us a capsule of pure fact.

Of course, fact has its value. Fact conveys a certain, limited information. Though we think of facts as true, facts alone cannot provide the kind of comprehensive knowledge that constitutes truth. There is none of this comprehensive truth in data. Fact is just fact, sterile, an empty vessel.

The newspaper tells us that what is important is the fact that there has been a car crash at the corner of 19th and Main Streets in which three persons have died. This piece of data cannot help us. It speaks only to a tiny part of us, our intellect and the most minimal range of our emotions. There is no life here. Worse, it depresses us. Is life then nothing more than a spectacular car crash? Are there no deeper, wider, richer experiences to look forward to? Were there no events today that might have made us feel glad to be alive?

The evening news: we are shown troops massing along both sides of a border. I watch footage of khaki colored tanks, jeeps, armored personnel carriers. A general, his weather-beaten face wary, stands before cameras on an expanse of sand. His rhetoric is confident. In his opinion, his men and materiel are superior. Our side will win.

The camera cuts to the next bit. This piece of data cannot help us. It speaks only to a tiny part of us, our intellect and the most minimal range of our emotions. Worse, it depresses us. There is no life here. This news is made to seem like a slice of life, but this is fakery. The general's words are not really his words. The general's words are rhetoric, what he thinks it is prudent to say in public.

In all three of these examples, statistics, journalism, and TV news coverage, we are asked to focus on the narrow, the minimal, the trivial, the gaudy, the grotesque, the grim, the sensational. We are asked to accept these things as important. We are not convinced. We know these pieces of data cannot help us. There is no life in them, and worse, they depress us. We go away anxious, our senses dulled. We go away hungry. We have been given only a piece of data, an empty vessel.

It is not a failure of data that the narrow range of fact it delivers is so limited. It is a failure of our culture that data is considered more important than story, because it is story and only story that conveys truth. We must have truth in order to arrive at wisdom, the power of judging rightly and following the soundest course of action.

I like the Nunamiut's definition of a storyteller. The storyteller is "the person who creates the atmosphere in which wisdom reveals itself."

A story is not a fantasy. It is not a glib, superficial ditty celebrating a life of bliss we never actually experience; nor is its opposite, the depressing news report of the car crash, a story. Both are slanted, both are one-sided. Both leave out the complexity of existence.

A story takes the measure of life with all its complexities. It reflects accurately a world we can recognize. "Our surroundings," Lopez (1990) writes, "are organized according to principles. . . . beyond human control" and contain "an integrity that is beyond human analysis and unimpeachable." These surroundings constitute our reality. Insofar as the storyteller depicts both the subtle and obvious relationships (in our surroundings) accurately, "the narrative will ring true" (Lopez, 1990, p. 66).

When you tell a story, you convey to another person the truth of a particular and unique situation as you experienced it. The resident's story rings true because it reflects a world we recognize. It is slanted neither toward unrealistic bliss nor toward unrealistic anguish. It contains elements of both bliss and anguish. If the patient playing with light were not dying, the story might seem merely anecdotal. It is the fact of the patient's imminent death that makes playing with the light a poignant and moving story. It rings true because we know our lives do not take place in a vacuum. Our lives take place in the context of mortality. Because the story reflects this crucial fact of our existence, it rings true.

Listen to another nurse's story (Krysl, 1989).

Sunshine Acres Living Center

The first thing you see up ahead is Mr.
Polanski, wedged in the
arched doorway, like he means absolutely
to stay there, he who shouldn't
be here in the first place, put in here
by mistake, courtesy of that grandson
who thinks himself a hotshot, and too busy
raking in the dough to find time for an old
man. If Polanski had anyplace
to go, he'd be out
instantly. If he had any

money. Which he doesn't, but he does have
a sharp eye, and intends to stay in that
doorway, not missing
a thing, and waiting
for trouble. Which of course
will come. And could be
you—you're handy, you look
likely, you have

the authority. And
you're new here, another young
whippersnapper, doesn't know
ass from elbow, but has been given
the keys. Well he's

ready, Polanski. *Mr. Polanski, good
morning*—you say it in Polish,
which you learned a little of
when you were little, and your grandmother
taught you a little song about lambs, frisking
in a pen, and you danced a silly little dance
with your grandmother, while the two of you
sang. So you sing it
for him, here in the dim, institutional
light of the hallway, light which even you
find insupportable, because even those who just
work here and can leave when their
shift ends deserve light to
see by, and because it reminds you
of the light in the hallway
outside the room
where, when your grandmother
died, you were three thousand miles

away. So that you're singing the little song
and remembering the silly little dance
to console yourself, and to pay your grandmother
tribute, and to try to charm Polanski,

which you do: you sing, and Mr. Polanski,
he who had set himself against the doorjamb
to resist you, he who had made of himself
a fist, Mr. Polanski,
    contentious, often
    combative and always
    and finally
    inconsolable
hears that you know
the song. And he steps out
from the battlement
of the doorway, and begins to
shuffle

and sing along.*

---

*Reprinted from M. Krysl (1989). *Midwife and Other Poems on Caring* (pp. 35–36). New York: National League for Nursing. Reprinted by permission.

This story details the complexity of life as we experience it. Polanski has a personality and a personal history. Polanski is difficult, contentious, combative because he does not want to be in the rest home. He directs his resentment toward the caregiver because she is an authority figure in the rest home and because at that moment, she's there, she's handy. The caregiver also has a personality and a personal history. She is drawn to Polanski because his Polish name reminds her of her grandmother and calls up the remorse she feels because she was not present at her grandmother's death. Because the caregiver has this personal history she is able, for a moment, to heal Polanski.

You who are caregivers understand that your contacts with patients do not take place in a vacuum. They take place in a rich context of personality and personal history and immediate, existential circumstances. Only story can convey this rich reality.

There is another reason story, not data, has the power to heal. We accept a piece of data for what it is: fact. It exists in tables or graphs or in the daily news. We go to tables, graphs, and the news when we want fact. Fact possesses no rich, authentic context which will bring it alive. It is just fact. It exists, if you will, in a vacuum.

The intense, vital, emotional energy of a story does not exist in a vacuum. Story is by its nature personal. It involves, always, at least two people. It cannot occur other than from person to person, from speaker to hearer, from writer to reader. It is by its very nature communal.

It is communal because when we tell a story, something happens to both the storyteller and the story-hearer.

What happens to the storyteller? When we tell a story, an intense energy wells up in us and flows out in speech or writing. An Eskimo man of the Netsalik group describes this.

> Man is moved just like the ice floe sailing here and there out in the current. His thoughts are driven by a flowing force when he feels joy, when he feels fear, when he feels sorrow. Thoughts can wash over him like a flood, making his breath come in gasps and his heart throb. And then it will happen

that we, who always think we are small, will feel still smaller. And we will fear to use words. But it will happen that the words we need will come of themselves. When the words we want shoot up of themselves—we get a new song.

"When the words we want shoot up of themselves." To tell a story is an act of vitality. It originates in the heart, and the story-teller herself is moved by her own telling. The telling uses not just her intellect and the most minimal range of her emotions. It uses all of her complex history leading up to this moment. It uses and energizes all of her, the whole person. She experiences "an inexplicable renewal of enthusiasm." She is buoyed up and her spirits lifted.

What happens to the hearer? The hearer hears not just with intellect and the most minimal range of emotions but as a whole person. The hearer too feels "an inexplicable renewal of enthusiasm." Story repairs our spirits. We feel buoyed up and our spirits are lifted.

Something happens to the storyteller and to the story-hearer. Something happens *between* them.

Consider for a moment the word *hearsay*. In our culture hearsay has no credibility. It connotes cheapness, triviality, mere gossip, rumor. All of these lack validity. We do not credit hearsay. Hearsay, however, also means report, and common talk. Report, common talk: that rich stream of communication between living persons, wealth without which human beings cannot live. The word hearsay richly describes what happens when we tell each other stories. I hear what you say, or you hear what I say. There is a speaker and a hearer, and between them there is reciprocity. Energy passes back and forth between them.

Feminist psychologist Ann Wilson Schaef describes love this way:

> An energy exchange that leaves the heart area of one person and enters the solar plexus of the other. It then moves up the body, that person takes some because she is loved and adds even more because one is loving. It then moves to the heart area and is sent back to the other.

When we love, energy flows out of us toward the beloved person and flows back from that person. I submit that when we tell a story, energy flows out of us toward the hearer and back from the hearer.

The resident who saw the woman playing with light says, "I noticed that some of my patients (people who had no education beyond high school, and a few not even that much) would keep repeating the lyrics of a song, or they would repeat a phrase they had heard in church—holding on for dear life to some words" (Coles, 1989, p. 100). What he was seeing was the way in which story, even a bit of a story, can feed us, heal us, keep us alive.

As Coles says, "What ought to be interesting . . . is the unfolding of a lived life rather than the confirmation such a chronicle provides for some theory." (Coles, 1989, p. 22)

Poet and physician William Carlos Williams reports the unfolding of the lived lives of his patients this way.

> Sometimes when I'm with a patient who is having trouble getting across to me what he wants to say, I tell him to stop describing the pain and just tell me where he was when the pain came on, and what he was doing. I say to him: 'When the pain knocked on your door, interrupting your life, what were you doing?' I try to get them to talk about that life before the interruption, and then as they describe the interruption, I can get a better picture of what happened than if they spend their time trying to find the right words for the bellyache or the chest pain.

Consider for a moment the anguish that results for us when our stories are not told. Levi (1961) reports a dream he dreamed repeatedly, in fact almost every night, during the time he was an inmate in Auschwitz.

In the dream Levi is back home in the presence of his family and friends, telling them of his experiences in Auschwitz.

> It is an intense pleasure, physical, inexpressible, to be at home, among friendly people, and to have so many things to recount, but I cannot help noticing that my listeners do not follow me. In fact, they are completely indifferent. They

speak confusedly of other things among themselves, as if I was not there. My sister looks at me, gets up and goes away without a word.

A desolating grief is now born in me, like certain barely remembered pains of one's early infancy. It is pain in its pure state, not tempered by a sense of reality and by the intrusion of extraneous circumstances, a pain like that which makes children cry. . . . I deliberately open my eyes, wake up. My dream stands in front of me, still warm, and although awake I am still full of its anguish. . . . [Levi, 1961]

It is a dream dreamed not only by Levi but by many other inmates of Auschwitz, possibly by all of them. Levi calls it the dream of the unlistened to story. Yet isn't this also the dream of how thwarted and unfulfilled we feel when we do not tell our stories?

When we do not tell our stories it is as though we create a death in ourselves by withholding, by not telling. We experience a loss, an impoverishment. Without our stories we are incomplete beings, stifled beings. We are patients in need of healing. Telling our stories heals us.

By not telling we also impoverish others. We withhold ourselves from others. We starve those we might feed.

A poem by 13th century ecstatic Persian poet Rumi, declares: "When a man or woman on the path refuses to praise, that man or woman is stealing from other people every day."

Stories are spiritual forces, like prayers. They can heal us and heal others. Our stories go out from us in widening circles. Those of us who live in white skins have been conditioned to discount the power of story. We would do well to learn of its power from our Native American brothers and sisters. American Indian people know stories have power both for good and for evil, depending on who uses them and for what purpose. In Silko's (1977) novel *Ceremony,* good and bad witches compete to see who can tell the best story.

One witch begins a story this way:

> Laugh if you want to
> but as I tell the story
> it will begin to happen.

He then tells the story of the coming of white people, how they will kill the animals, poison the water, slaughter whole tribes, bring disease and eventually destroy everything, including themselves.

The others concede his story wins the prize. But they want him to rescind his story.

> What you said just now—
> it isn't so funny
> It doesn't sound so good.
> We are doing okay without it
> We can get along without that kind of thing.
> Take it back
> Call that story back.
> The witch replies:
> It's already turned loose
> It's already coming
> It can't be called back   [Silko, 1977]

The witch's story can only be prevented from happening by telling a more powerful story. Good stories can't be called back either. Stories are spiritual forces like prayers—or as Rumi wrote, "everything has to do with loving or not loving." Not to tell our story is to give in to the witch's story. Not to tell our story is to acquiesce to the dominant story in which we are now living.

Writer James Baldwin said of his early life as a black child in America: "Growing up in a certain kind of poverty is growing up in a certain kind of silence." He said that inside that silence you cannot name the sensations, fears, injustices, and simple facts of daily life because "no one corroborates it. Reality becomes unreal because no one experiences it but you." When the young Baldwin read the work of his predecessor, Richard Wright, he felt that "life was made bearable by Richard Wright's testimony. When circumstances are made real by another's testimony, it becomes possible to envision change."

Storytellers are in fact our best guarantee against any kind of totalitarianism. Only if we do not lie, only if we report what happens accurately and in all its complex detail, only then can we know what is truly happening, and only then can we act with wisdom.

Lopez (1990) writes that ". . . truth reveals itself most fully not in dogma, but in paradox, irony and contradictions . . . beyond this there are only failures of imagination; reductionism in science; fundamentalism in religion; fanaticism in politics."

"The stories people tell have a way of taking care of them," Lopez writes. "If stories come to you, care for them. And learn to give them away when they are needed. Sometimes a person needs a story more than food to stay alive. That is why we put these stories in each other's memory. This is how people care for themselves" (Lopez, 1990).

REFERENCES

Coles, R. (1989). *The call of stories: Teaching and the moral imagination.* Boston: Houghton Mifflin.

Krysl, M. (1989). *Midwife and other poems on caring.* New York: National League for Nursing.

Levi, P. (1961). *Survival at Auschwitz.* New York: Macmillan.

Lopez, B. (1990). *Crow and weasel.* Berkeley: North Point Press.

Silko, L. (1977). *Ceremony.* New York: Penguin.

4

The Emancipatory Power of the Narrative

Nancy Diekelmann

EMPOWERING NARRATIVES: OUR STORIES/OUR SELVES

Our stories of teaching—of the times we will never forget because they speak of what it means to be a teacher in nursing—tell of times of breakdown, when nothing went right, and times of connectedness, when we made a difference as a teacher. These are empowering narratives because they reveal our expertise as teachers. They make visible the *how* of nursing education. Patricia Benner (1984; Benner & Wrubel, 1989) has shown that the stories of nurses reveal both the evolution and nature of nursing practice. They also reveal the practical knowledge that is embedded in nursing practice as it develops over time. Our stories of teaching reveal our expertise, our dilemmas, and our practical knowledge. These are emancipatory narratives because they recognize our expertise, help us to know each other, transform our thinking, and help us in creating communities.

41

RECOGNIZING TEACHER EXPERTISE

Relating these narratives empowers us as we strive to uncover and reveal to ourselves the level of expertise in our own practice. This mode of scholarship can be a helpful guide as we struggle to transform our teaching.

As we listen to our stories, we realize that many of the dilemmas and experiences they articulate are similar; what emerges are our common understandings and the shared practices of teaching. For example, one such shared practice is "getting through to a student." We have all as teachers had students who we worked hard at trying "to get through to." This "getting through" is difficult to describe acontextually, or to teach to a new nurse teacher. It is not a unidirectional "getting through"; rather it is working toward a Gadamerian fusion of horizons (Gadamer, 1960/1989). It is a common practice that we all share, and is best revealed in a specific context, a story, as this story by Pam Scheibel demonstrates.

"Getting Through to the Student"

I was a clinical instructor on a cardiac floor where most of the patients were either a stepdown from the CCU or on observation to go to the CCU, CC list, or surgery. These senior students were somewhat anxious about the care of these kinds of patients, but one student was particularly anxious. She would *over read* and *over worry* about her patients. She would see the *zebras in the forest* always thinking the worse case scenarios! I tried regularly to talk about her anxiety with her. She always agreed she was too anxious and was trying to change. I was at wits end trying to think of a way to get the student to decrease her anxiety and "lighten up" on herself. I knew she had the knowledge necessary to make the right decisions regarding patient care, but my constant reminding her to slow down, look at the information logically and process it correctly, without the anxiety she exhibited, bothered me. One day near the end of the semester I was struggling with myself regarding her. I remember sitting at the nurses' station with my hand over my mouth when this student came up to me and said in her usual anxious, almost hysterical way, "My patient

Mr. W. who had a suspected M.I., his enzymes are 3,000!" I looked at this incredibly caring, intelligent student with my hand on my mouth and decided to take a chance. I moved my hand down to my chin and I said, in a calm and almost humorous voice, "Uh, I can't remember, is that high or low?" The student stopped breathing for a moment as she looked at my face and I at her, my hand once more over my mouth. Suddenly I noticed she relaxed the muscles I could see, and she smiled and said "High" and a moment later, "Thank you." I received a Christmas card from that student the following year. She signed it "High!—Susan."

Teaching is not without its risks. This vignette tells of a teacher taking a risk to "get through to" an overly anxious student. In the struggle of how to reach this student, this teacher knows that these words will be interpreted by the student as ridicule if not said just right. But the timing was good: the teacher connected with this student. Making contact or "getting through" to students is a shared practice of teaching. It is what teaching is all about.

As experienced teachers, we all know what "getting through" to a student means, and we know when we have done it. Yet it is a part of our practice of teaching that is invisible to new teachers. We try to capture this part of our practice when we use such terms as "the teachable moment." Yet, this sense of timing, knowing when and how to intervene as we seek to get through to the student, is a common practice that we share and is best revealed through sharing our stories. Knowledge of when and how to "get through" is developed over time, and the skill is obtained by getting it wrong a lot of times before one begins to get one's timing right.

KNOWING THE STUDENT—KNOWING EACH OTHER

Knowing the patient is a hallmark of nursing care (Benner & Tanner, 1987). Knowing the student is also central to the practice of teaching. As nurse teachers we often go to great lengths to get to know students. It is not easy in large classes, but we work creatively to find ways and assignments that help us get to know our students. We also work hard to find ways our students can get to know us. Finding the right level of involvement, and the boundaries of our practice of teaching, happens over time. It is through getting it wrong, becoming over and underinvolved, that one finally begins getting the right level of involvement enabling the teacher to move closer to knowing students.

The paradox is that while we spend a lot of time getting to know our students, we do not always see the importance of, or know how to get, the same right level of involvement with our teaching colleagues. Because we see each other so much, we think we know each other. Telling our stories of teaching can help us to know each other in new ways. Our colleagues' stories can reveal a part of them and their teaching practice that we rarely see. How easy it is for us to talk about our problems in teaching. In point of fact, however, it is difficult for us to talk about our successes without feeling like we are bragging.

A new director of a nursing school decided that the faculty should each take three minutes to tell everyone what they had accomplished in the last year. She related that:

> I thought this would be helpful for me getting to know the faculty and them getting to know each other. I had to do merit reviews and I had all this information they had submitted on what they had done and I was amazed! My faculty was an incredibly talented, creative, and productive group. What I began discovering was that they didn't tell each other what they were doing or accomplishing. So I had this bright idea of taking three minutes once a year as a part of our end of the year faculty meeting. . . . Well, what a disaster. I had faculty come to me and say, "I won't come if we have to do 'Show and Tell.'" Another said, "It's nobody's business what consulting or writing I do during the year." And then there was the new faculty who felt like they were being put on the spot because "all" they had done was teach their courses. So I dropped the idea, but I still think it is a good one.

This story revealed how the practice of describing what was accomplished during the year, and what had been meaningful for faculty, became a competitive, highly stressful experience. When this practice is described as "show and tell," it makes impossible a simple experience that could help teachers in knowing one another. The practice of calling this "show and tell" perpetuates teacher isolation and encourages faculty not to know each other as opposed to creating communities of care in teaching (Bellah, Madsen, Sullivan, Swidler, & Tipton, 1985). Sandie Soldwisch, a new PhD and assistant professor, described another kind of teacher isolation:

> [Creative teaching] already takes up so much of my time and I have family pressures like most everyone else in the world has family pressures. But then I also have the pressures of trying to meet a tenure requirement, learning how to do publishing, trying to establish a network of people who know that I even exist, so that somewhere along the line they will ask me to submit abstracts or presentations. I don't know how to go about all of that . . . I don't know where I should have learned it, but I didn't learn it. So now I'm learning it on my own, which is OK, but it's taking up an awful lot of very valuable tenure time . . . and . . . I think that we should have more of a collegial feeling . . . and since I do not have a colleagueship, there's no one there to say to me, "well that idea sounds great but have you ever thought of such and such?" Now, if I can't find the time to do the publishing and the research and the consulting and the presentations, I don't know how I'd find the time to develop this colleagueship either. I feel a tremendous need for something of this nature.

This narrative resonates loudly for those of us involved directly in doctoral education and teacher preparation. Where do you learn how to bring your scholarship and teaching practices together in ways so they do not compete? Typically doctoral students have had or take coursework in teaching and perhaps even a teaching practicum, or gain teaching experience as a teaching assistant. But where do they learn the *invisible part of our practices?* Through narratives, experienced nurse teachers can begin to reveal how they learned to secrete away a day to write or do research.

For instance, experienced teachers have learned it is important to their research that they teach the same course over and over. They realize that the only people who should be taking a new course every semester are students—not teachers. However, the understanding that it is important to insist on stability in teaching assignments in order to know a course well enough to have time to do research and writing, is often only afforded to faculty *after* they are tenured, when they least need it. The emancipatory power of the narrative is in not just revealing these practices to us, but in helping us see how we need to overcome and transform the situations that perpetuate oppression and powerlessness.

How could we, in the context of schooling, help better prepare PhD students for the practice of teaching and research? How can we as senior faculty reflect on our own teaching so that we are aware how important stable assignments for tenure-bound faculty are, and thus create schools and curricula that attend to this dilemma? My research reveals it is only when a teacher has had a course long enough to know it, that the teacher can move from teacher to learner. *To learn a course, you first teach it.* This is a curious paradox, and one for us to reflect upon. How do we decide who will teach what course and when? The constant learning of new courses, the lack of collegial guidance, and the competition for time, all contribute to teacher isolation.

TEACHING AS A WAY OF THINKING

Embedded within our stories are our shared understandings of how we approach, participate in, and experience thinking in teaching nursing. There are many possible paths in thinking. Thinking as a pathway does not necessarily lead to a predetermined outcome (Heidegger, 1954/1968, 1959/1966). Among possible pathways are: Nursing As a Way of Thinking (Rather, 1990) and Teaching as Learning (Diekelmann, 1990).

Heidegger (1954/1968) has asserted that:

> we are still not thinking . . . although the state of the world
> is becoming constantly more thought-provoking (p. 4).

For me, this curriculum revolution is characterized by *an explication of how we think*. Most of the changes in previous educational reforms have been characterized by new curricular or organizational approaches to courses and course content, or by new instructional approaches to teaching and learning. My research points to the need to focus not on curriculum or instruction but on how we think about the common everyday problems that confront us.

Consider the genius of Frank Lloyd Wright. We can use his work to realize that the worlds of science and aesthetics have been traditionally experienced as discrete parts of thinking by the modern tradition. Heidegger (1954/1968) explicated this idea of the world in terms of what he thought to be closer to its essential structuring. He wrote:

> In so far as we caringly hold thing as thing, we dwell in the near. Nearing of the near is the genuine and unique dimension of the mirror-play of the world (p. 18, translation modified).

The practice of architecture is another path to thinking. The drawings of Frank Lloyd Wright, admired as they are for their beauty, are important records of his practice. While he displayed these drawings for pleasure and instruction, he saw them not as some linear exploration of alternatives or conceptual acrobatics, but rather as reflections of his work on the fluid integration of space and structure. His thinking about house and home was in a context that sought to understand the meaning of habitation, to inspire people, to excite them but not to disturb them.

Another renowned architect, Ludwig Mies van der Rohe (1946) described the work of Frank Lloyd Wright as an architectural world whose dynamic impulse, clarity of language, and exuberant richness of form invigorated a whole generation of young architects.

In some respects the work of Frank Lloyd Wright reflected the energy and egalitarianism that described the United States of the turn of the century. His justly famed residential work maintained the hearth as a dwelling's spiritual center, while doing away with the boxlike rooms of that time (Wright, 1954). He developed plans with interpenetrating spaces and worked to integrate the exterior and interior worlds of the buildings' dwellers.

His surface decorative treatments were meant to symbolize the varied interrelationships and fecundity of nonhuman nature. Indigenous stone, horizontal roof lines, and large overhangs were attempts to evoke the physical features of a building's location. Frank Lloyd Wright's works were an attempt to develop what he called an organic architecture whose aesthetic symbolized fusion rather than separation or isolation. His works represented such Enlightenment ideals as rationality, democracy, progress, and freedom.

Hans George Gadamer (1960/1989) has asked us to look further at these ideals as they are a part of aesthetics as subjectivization. He states that "Nineteenth-century aesthetics was founded on the freedom of the symbol-making activity of the mind" (p. 81). Like Heidegger (1927/1962) before him, Gadamer questions whether this tradition of Cartesian representation can ever be a sufficient foundation for thinking.

The abstraction inherent in aesthetic experience stems from the separation of science as truth from art as autonomous example of "pure perception" (Gadamer, 1960/1989, p. 91). Gadamer attempts to retrieve the revealing nature of the work of art in his discussion of play. The being of the work of art involves a complex of phenomena "at play" with one another.

Despite the genius and brilliance that marks the achievement of Taliesin West, it is still a house in a hot, dry environment with its artificially irrigated lawns, shrubs, and trees. For all of its use of indigenous materials, its symbolic representations do little to reveal our relationships with nature. It is, in its own way, part of the tradition of disinterested knowledge that emphasizes the inert over entities that are freed for their own being (Heidegger 1927/1962, 1979/1985).

Little of Arizona's Sonoran desert remains that has not been radically affected by human activities. An area of high heat and low rainfall is not a desert. As a natural community, a desert is made up of the complex interaction of hundreds of different animals and plants with their physical environment.

Thinking is not a theoretical application of knowledge or a passive experience of reflection, like gazing at an art object. Thinking is dwelling in the world; a moving into nearness with what is near to us. We can view Taliesin West as a scientific architectural endeavor or as an aesthetic experience. We are dwelling in the world thinkingly when we experience Taliesin West as an afternoon with colleagues in which we are open and discuss the meaning of what shows up for us. It will be what we bring to the experience that will shape our path of thinking.

The thinking of teachers is revealed through their stories. Experienced teachers' stories often move from occasions when they reached students and made a difference, to times when they learned something about the meaning of learning from students. The structured language of teaching falls away and the hermeneutic language of learning emerges. Experienced teachers describe, even as they review old paradigms, times when they have learned from their experiences. The commitment to learning, both their own and others', becomes central to their conversations.

Shared practices, common meanings, and constitutive patterns in the teaching of nursing emerge through the use of Heideggerian hermeneutic explication (Diekelmann, Allen, & Tanner, 1989). My research (Diekelmann, In Press) on the lived experiences of teachers in nursing has revealed the following three patterns:

1. Changing *the* world, changing *my* world,
2. the teacher as learner, and
3. the learner as teacher.

Changing the World—Changing my World

Hubert Dreyfus (1991) has written that Heidegger's "description of the world as having a distinctive structure of its own that makes possible and calls forth" human ways of being is the "most important and original contribution of *Being and Time.*" We both *are* a world and *have* a world. The disclosure of shared patterns of commitments to make the world a better place occurs among students, new nurses, and new teachers.[1] Several teachers, in describing what it was like for them when they went into teaching, talked about how they wanted to teach differently than they were taught, and about how they wanted to prepare nurses to change nursing practice. Many teachers, in discussing the problems they had, began to see these practices from a new perspective. One teacher told me:

> I remember as a student nurse, being so afraid before clinical that I wouldn't sleep and I was almost sleep deprived by the end of the week. When I became a clinical instructor I worked hard to relieve the fears of my students until one day I heard one student say to another that she gets diarrhea before my clinical because she is so afraid. What I've learned is that the students will be afraid no matter what you do. Their fear has more to do with it being scary to care for such ill patients when you have little knowledge and experience than it does supportive teachers.

This teacher initially struggled to make the world of the entering student less fearful. Experience transformed this teacher's thinking.

> What I now do is talk to the students about the kind of back-up and protection we surround them with. In fact, to practice nursing is to care about your patients and protect them from inexperienced nurses and errors that anyone can make. I show them which patients I don't assign them and why. And I tell them that nurses will be checking up on them even when they don't know it by reading their charting, looking into their rooms when they are caring for their patients, and being sure that certain things get done at a certain time. You know, I just spend a lot of time showing them all the back-up that we give each other. That way they don't misinterpret our checking up on them. But also we talk about "nursing in the

---

[1]This pattern first emerged in a study by Marsha Rather (1990) on the lived experiences of returning registered nursing students as they talked about how their thinking had been transformed as a result of their experiences in practice. They found they no longer thought as they did when they were students in their basic nursing program.

dark" and how it feels to take care of patients when you are beginning, or anytime when you aren't sure you know all that you need to know. Nursing is dangerous in places—no?

The nurse thinks about the students' fears differently now. Rather than trying to reduce their fear, the teacher has learned to engage them in talking about their fears and what can be done about them. She says:

> I still don't understand all that students are afraid of, but I am learning an awful lot about what it means to be a student and afraid . . . that is helping me better understand. My focus now is not so much on being supportive as on trying to understand. It seems like this is the best kind of support I can give. Do you get what I am trying to say?

The issue is not what can we do as teachers to make students less fearful, but what it is about caring for patients that makes student nurses afraid. Trying to understand this dilemma can make a great difference in how teachers think about teaching clinical nursing.

This shift in thinking is subtle. Teaching as a way of thinking is situational, fluid, and transformative. It is hermeneutical. Hermeneutical thinking does not rush in but rather seeks to understand. The commitment is to explication, not to some form of critique.

Teaching is neither passive nor without critique; the central concern of this path is understanding. The teacher in the previous example did not focus on all the interventions that are possible to reduce the students' fear, but sought to learn the meaning of fear as a constitutive part of entering nursing practice. The teacher thought about the role of "being afraid" in novice nursing practice and how novice practice is shaped and informed by "being afraid," particularly the fear of doing harm to patients.

The change in the teacher's relationships with students also changed from a "leaping in" position of helping students to one of "leaping ahead" (Heidegger, 1927/1962). The teacher attended and bore witness to their fears, avoiding undue or excessive interventions.

A student brought this story into my class to describe this way of behavior.

> A nurse was walking along a path and came to a river and saw a person drowning. She jumped in and pulled the person out, started CPR and revived the person. Just then she looked up and saw another person drowning in the same spot. [She] Pulled the person out, started CPR, revived him, looked up and another person was drowning. [She] Jumped in, pulled the person out, started CPR, revived him and looked up and another person was drowning. As she jumped in this time, she started to think, *"I wonder what is going on upstream?"*

Our stories help us to know when and how to "leap in," but they also speak of looking "upstream" to try to understand what constitutes our concerns. We need to speak of the fears students have about making mistakes and failing in nursing and how we as teachers can help students deal with these fears in ways that do not immobilize them, but rather help them develop coping skills. We also need to look upstream and learn about the patterns of novice nursing practice—one pattern being the "proving ground" (Suchomel, 1987). The proving ground is a trial by ordeal for novice nurses. It is a proving to self and others that one can safely practice in nursing, assess dangerousness and seek out and use back-up. An important part of the proving ground is learning the boundaries of practice. We need to explore the boundaries of novice nursing care at a time when more patients are critically ill. We must reflect on how this acuity level is experienced by teachers, students, and clinicians.

The Teacher As Learner

The teacher as learner is another constitutive pattern that emerges in the stories of teachers in nursing. In these stories, teachers show what they learn from their students. Freire (1968/1970) describes the theme of teacher as learner as central to deconstructing the power relationships between students and teachers. The need for teachers to attend to their relationships with students was revealed when Shor (1986) wrote of students on strike, using the only means they had: passive resistance, suspiciousness, and lack of trust.

Many teachers work hard to find ways to minimize the power they have over students, but not all teachers do this. Thus, part of the curriculum revolution is to look at how our practices, though we intend otherwise, perpetuate the power we have over students and clinicians in nursing education.

A continuing concern of the curriculum revolution is to encourage all voices to join in our conversations. It must be of issue for us that there are not numbers of students joining our education conferences. We must reach out to our clinical colleagues and invite them to join us in this educational reform movement. Patients—the consumers of our care—and physicians need to have a place in this movement. How can we bring all these voices into our conversations about nursing education? With our past in front of us, we must together seek to engender egalitarian, pluralistic conversations to enable us to learn from each other.

The Learner As Teacher

The final constitutive pattern that emerged from the stories of nurse teachers is: the learner as teacher. In the previous section, I discussed how teachers continue to learn in their teaching practices. In this pattern, I will speak of how teachers come to know there is no such thing as teaching—only learning. That is, my analysis has revealed that the ontological nature of teaching is learning. Teaching is a special kind of learning, just as research as scholarship (Heidegger, 1950/1977) is a special kind of learning. *The practice of teaching is learning.* An experienced teacher used a maxim to describe his practice of teaching. He said:

> The more I teach, the more I realize that the less I teach, the more students learn. It's weird, but I am a better teacher now and I do half the teaching things I used to do—like reams of care plans and papers and checking up to see that students aren't falling behind and stuff like that. I just now only focus on how they are learning. I didn't realize it until the other day

when I was going through some of my old course syllabi from another school. . . . I really kept the students—and myself, I would add—very, very, very busy. I don't need to do so much teaching now because I understand learning.

Learning has a centrality in the practice of teaching nursing. Just as caring is central to nursing (Benner & Wrubel, 1989), learning is central to teaching (Heidegger, 1954/1968). This understanding of learning is primordial and ontological. It is a learning to let learn. Heidegger speaks of how teaching in this way becomes a special kind of learning.

> Teaching is even more difficult than learning. We know that, but we rarely think about it. And why is teaching more difficult than learning? Not because the teacher must have a larger store of information, and have it always ready. Teaching is more difficult than learning because what teaching calls for is this: *to let learn* [emphasis added]. The real teacher, in fact, lets nothing else be learned than—learning. His [*sic*] conduct, therefore, often produces the impression that we properly learn nothing from him, if by "learning" we now suddenly understand merely the procurement of useful information. The teacher is ahead of his apprentices in this alone, that he has still far more to learn than they—he has *to learn to let them learn. The teacher must be capable of being more teachable than the apprentices* [emphasis added]. The teacher is far less assured of his ground than those who learn are of theirs. If the relation between the teacher and the taught is genuine, therefore, there is never a place in it for the authority of the know-it-all of the authoritative sway of the official (Heidegger, 1954/1968, p. 15).

If it is learning that grounds us, then we must discuss those practices in teaching that encourage learning and those that make learning possible or impossible. We must reflect on how spending too much time evaluating or trying to organize the curriculum leaves little time to think and learn as a teacher. Do we create a place in our week to not just go to the library to look something up, but also to *dwell?* Is there a place for us to just look at all the new periodicals? Do we take the time we need to sit in on a colleague's course or a series of lectures at the university, or do we say, "I have papers to grade"?

Learning is reciprocal and the learner as teacher dwells in a community of care. One teacher told me this story about how her students cared for her as a learner:

> I teach a fundamentals course and we have a big end-of-the-quarter skills exam. Well, I wanted so much to go to this conference on physical assessment skills and, of course, it was during the week of our skills exams, when I'm really nuts trying to find time to test all the students. One day at the end of a class I mentioned this conference and said I really wished I could go, but you know. Well, two weeks later, at the beginning of lab, the students presented me with a schedule of three evenings the week before when they would be willing to have me test them in advance so I could go to the conference. I was so touched, I had tears in my eyes. One of the older students said to me, "You know the nicest thing about this is not that you appreciate what we've done, but that you confided in us so we could care for you—a teacher—for a change. I always have the feeling around this school that the teachers are supposed to care about the students, but the students aren't supposed to care about the teachers."

Later, the teacher concluded this story with the statement, "The more I teach, the more I learn, and learn that learning is all we can ever do."

First as nurses, and later as teachers of nursing, we know how important *to be able to give caring* is to sustaining life. Doing the least amount possible in our practice with students and patients is a form our care takes not because we are lazy and withholding, but rather because we understand how important reciprocity is in sustaining the human experience through care. Yet we make it difficult if not impossible for our colleagues and students to care for us. Many teachers speak of their weariness in coping with times of poor resources, increasing acuity levels with patients, and staff shortages. It makes care and teaching very difficult. Yet the need is great for reciprocity; for us to show how, in order to have the caring communities we need to sustain us, we need both people who care and people we are willing to be cared for.

Reciprocity as a constitutive part of caring, i.e., we need both to care and to be cared for in order for caring communities to exist, is an important conversation for us to have. We can seek to talk about the caring we give and the caring we receive. We can share with one another and become comfortable with conversations that are personal and speak of our lived experiences.

A NEW WAY OF THINKING—UNVEILING INNOVATION

For me this revolution is at hand. As I hear the stories of teachers, students, and clinicians, I have discovered that there is innovation everywhere. The changes are simple and at hand and at the same time complex and impossible.

Our stories are simple, yet profound. Heidegger (1947/1971) describes this possibility as the splendor of the simple. Our stories are full of simple and complex possibilities to transform our practice of teaching as learning. I have come to realize that some of the difficulty we experience stems from the fact that we seek change as innovation; innovation as something new or untried, or never heard of before. As we share our stories with one another, I propose we create a place for a new way of thinking about innovation.

Our experience and our tradition in nursing education is to consider something innovative as having the characteristic of being new and unfamiliar to us as teachers. We discount approaches if we are using them, or have successfully used them. There is a tendency to conclude that nothing innovative could be familiar or used successfully in the past or in other contexts. We ask: how would I know an innovative approach to teaching, learning, or curriculum if I saw or heard one?

Missing from this approach to thinking about innovation is that it may be in the familiar, the reflecting on what we currently do successfully, that innovation in our current practice will arise. To think of innovation as something new from an outside source rules out the possibility that innovation resides and arises from our own experience (way of being) (Gadamer, 1960/1989). It covers over and reduces to the trivial the innovations one has currently embraced. This view of innovation as coming from the other—a consultant, or an expert, or a researcher—de-skills us and encourages us to believe we neither know what we are doing nor how to create a future of innovation and new possibilities (Diekelmann, 1991). Let us listen to how a teacher described an experience with innovation in nursing education:

> I want to tell you about this Med-Surg course I teach. I had been teaching it for nine years when I decided I wanted to do something different, innovative. You know how you get bored and stuff. . . . there are usually six or seven other faculty in and out of the course with me taking clinical sections. Well, we had this clinical evaluation tool. I mean it was good. Both valid and reliable and we had worked for years on getting it down pat. . . . I said to them, this was over three years ago, look if you don't want to use this tool, *don't*. If it helps you do, but if you want to adapt it or improve [it] or use something else or another approach, *do*. I still to this day don't know why I did that, but I did. Actually I do. I was tired of hearing how much time faculty were spending on anecdotal notes and filling out the tool. Some of the instructors said they were spending almost 45 minutes each week on filling out the tool. It had gotten to be five full pages . . . I wanted to make it easier on both the students and the teachers. So I thought let's be innovative . . . the first year it was real difficult with my faculty. As lead instructor, I was used to working with them around student problems . . . but suddenly, I was being asked like permission, if it was OK to change the teaching-learning project objectives in the tool and . . . I said sure, that's what I meant about adapting the tool. . . . Another teacher looked like she wasn't going to use anything and then at the last minute had a real hard time, and I had to kind of bail her out. I think she was testing me. I was almost tempted to go back to the consistent tool— believe me. But I didn't. The faculty had to know that I believed that they could best decide how to evaluate their students . . . somehow I knew we had lost something when we became so consistent. Anyway, back to my story. The next two semesters it was worse. The teachers finally believed me

and each of them were doing their own thing. But the students were furious. They kept coming to me with complaints of "Mrs. So and So doesn't require a patient teaching project and my instructor does. That's not fair." And I would talk to them about focusing on what is important about patient teaching with their patients . . . not what others in the course are doing or not doing, but on what it is like for them with their instructor with their patients in their section of the course. For a while it was tough . . . until now where the students understand that overall objectives for the courses are the same, but each instructor develops approaches to meeting and evaluating the course given a particular clinical population. But the ending of all this is the best. I for the first time have seen this course go from a "killer" course—I didn't tell you the students used to hate it—to the course with consistently the highest student evaluations! There were years where no one wanted to teach in my course because there was so much content and it was so hard and now I have faculty requesting a section in my course—do you believe it? And quite honestly, the only thing I changed was our use of our clinical tool! I wished I had thought of it before!

Innovation can be as near as a change in our thinking. The previous story speaks of the power and splendor of the simple. The changing of something as simple as the practice of using the same grading tool led to the emerging of new possibilities that transformed the learning situation. As we reflect on our stories, we open up new ways of thinking about many of the practices that we have taken for granted, e.g., using a consistent tool in a course.

One wonders, then what do our colleagues in neighboring offices have to show us abut innovation? Does the teacher in the next office view the transformation of the course as finally getting clinical assignments that are meaningful? Perhaps finding a good textbook was the reason student evaluations of the course changed. Or might one think that the teacher mellowed or became easier to work with, or was "made" to stop being so rigid as a result of negative student evaluations of the course? Narratives help us to know each other from the inside out. Viewing the course situation from the outside, the previous interpretations are all possible. It is only when we hear the story that we understand the change in the lead teacher's thinking about consistency and fairness. What the story made visible is the teacher's insight and skill in effecting the transition from a structured to a revisioned course. This teacher minimized effecting and participating in this change, but one cannot help but see the skill and sensitivity brought to the situation. As we create a place for new conversations between students and teachers, and between teachers and teachers, this paradigm points to a powerful understanding of "teaching as a way of thinking."

CREATING COMMUNITIES OF CARE

The curriculum revolution is a way of unveiling new approaches, programs, and ideas which can inform and change current curricular and instructional practices in our schools of nursing. We need to set up networks within our regions to share and support the innovation and reform we are creating and re-creating in our schools. We are greatly enhanced by sharing our experiences in an era of plurality in educational programs. The development of cohort groups is a step toward creating regional conversations.

Our stories, our experiences with innovation, are instructive and supportive. Of primary importance is the development of an empowering new literature for nursing teachers, students, and clinicians.

As teachers describe their day-to-day experiences, I am amazed by the isolation that emerges. Teachers see each other with regularity and spend large parts of their days in meetings and talking to each other. What I have begun to realize, however, is that the majority of this time is often spent on such activities as solving problems, fighting over policies or procedures, or competing over resources. It is no wonder that we do not get to know each other, and feel isolated. The danger lies in the fact that some of the isolation we experience is greatest when we *do not* feel removed or isolated because we spend so much time together (Michelfelder & Palmer, 1989).

The meaning of isolation is not *knowing* your colleagues. We must begin to practice new conversations, new ways of speaking to each other, so we come to know each other. These ought not to be the abstract or theoretical conversations that perpetuate the competition and isolation we feel. Our stories *are* the conversations of our experiences in which we come to know one another.

Creating communities will also lead us into conversations about caring. Because we seek to create communities of care and responsibility, we must reflect on the reciprocity of caring. How do we care for students and clinicians, ourselves and fellow teaching colleagues? How do we teach caring for patients? How can we create communities of care when we have colleagues who are destructive and unable to accept or give caringly?

Lastly, how can we transform our thinking? Perhaps a transformation we will all share will be to move away from our insistence on goals or outcomes or even on accomplishing the revolution. Verle Waters asked me if I thought I would live long enough to see a curriculum revolution or the reforms we speak of today implemented. My response was that it really did not concern me that we accomplish this end, or any end in view. What matters to me is that I will spend the rest of my professional life trying to transform nursing education. I seek to be a teacher as learner, and a learner as teacher, and to get better and better at being in the stream, ever mindful of the thinking necessary to understand what is going on upstream. I invite you to participate in sharing your stories of teaching as we create and re-create our future through the emancipatory power of the narrative.

REFERENCES

Bellah, N., Madsen, R., Sullivan, W., Swidler, A., & Tipton, S. (1985). *Habits of the heart: Individualism and commitment in American life.* New York: Harper & Row.

Benner, P. (1984). *From novice to expert: Excellence and power in clinical nursing practice.* Menlo Park, CA: Addison-Wesley.

Benner, P., & Tanner, C. (1987). Clinical judgment: How expert nurses use intuition. *American Journal of Nursing, 87*(1), 23–31.

Benner, P., & Wrubel, J. (1989). *The primacy of caring: Stress and coping in health and illness.* Menlo Park, CA: Addison-Wesley.

Diekelmann, N. (1990). Nursing education: Caring, dialogue, and practice. *Journal of Nursing Education, 29*(7), 300–305.

Diekelmann, N. (1991, January). *Nursing education: Caring, dialogue, and practice: Hermeneutic experience as inquiry.* Paper presented at 23rd Open Seminar for Nurse Scholars, Tokyo, Japan.

Diekelmann, N. (In Press). Nursing education: Caring, dialogue and practice. New York: National League for Nursing.

Diekelmann, N., Allen, D., & Tanner, C. (1989). *The NLN criteria for appraisal of baccalaureate programs: A critical hermeneutic analysis.* New York: National League for Nursing.

Dreyfus, H. (1991). *Being-in-the-world: A commentary on Heidegger's Being and Time, Division 1.* Cambridge, MA: MIT Press.

Freire, P. (1970). *Pedagogy of the oppressed* (M. Ramos, Trans.). New York: The Continuum Publishing Corp. (Original work published 1968/1970)

Gadamer, H. G. (1989). *Truth and method* (2nd revised ed.) (J. Weinsheimer & D. Marshall, Trans.). New York: The Crossroad Publishing Co. (Original work published 1960)

Heidegger, M. (1962). *Being and time* (J. Macquarrie & E. Robinson, Trans.). New York: Harper & Row. (Original work published 1927)

Heidegger, M. (1966). *Discourse on thinking* (J. Anderson & E. H. Freund, Trans.). New York: Harper & Row. (Original work published 1959)

Heidegger, M. (1968). *What is called thinking?* (F. Wieck & J. Gray, Trans.). New York: Harper & Row. (Original work published 1954)

Heidegger, M. (1971). The thinker as poet. In *Poetry, language, thought* (pp. 1–14) (A. Hofstadter, Trans.). New York: Harper & Row. (Original work published 1947)

Heidegger, M. (1977). The age of the world picture. In *The question concerning technology and other essays* (W. Lovitt, Trans.). New York: Harper & Row. (Original work published 1950)

Heidegger, M. (1985). *History of the concept of time.* (T. Kisiel, Trans.). Bloomington: Indiana University Press. (Original work published 1979)

Heidegger, M. (1990). The thing. In *Poetry, language, thought* (pp. 163–186) (A. Hofstadter, Trans.). New York: Harper & Row. (Original work published 1954)

Michelfelder, D., & Palmer, R. (1989). *Dialogue and deconstruction: The Gadamer–Derrida encounter.* Albany, NY: State University of New York Press.

Mies van der Rohe, L. (1946, autumn). A tribute to Frank Lloyd Wright. *College Art Journal, 6*(1), 41-2.

Rather, M. (1990). The lived experience of returning registered nurse students: A Heideggerian hermeneutical analysis (Doctoral dissertation, University of Wisconsin–Madison, 1990). University Microfilms No. 90-24783.

Shor, I. (1986). *Cultural wars: School and society in the conservative restoration, 1969–1984.* London: Routledge & Kegan Paul.

Suchomel, S. (1987). *The novice nurse entry into critical care nursing practice: Socialization and evolution of clinical judgment-making.* Unpublished master's thesis, University of Wisconsin-Madison, Madison, WI.

Wright, F. (1954). *The natural house.* New York: Bramhall Press.

5

Alice in Wonderland: A Metaphor for Professional Nursing Education

Susan S. Gunby,
Pamela Chally,
Regina E. Dorman,
Kathryn M. Grams,
Margaret M. Kosowski, and
Betsy S. Pless

A dilemma exists within the curriculum revolution in nursing. At a time when the trend is toward broader nondisciplinary education, professional nurse educators are striving to clarify the experiences of nurses in higher education, as well as to justify to the profession and the health care delivery system the competence of nursing graduates. The pull at both ends of the continuum, from broad-based liberal education at one end to criteria-based professional education at the other, creates a dichotomy for educators who are never able to satisfactorily serve both masters.

Modes of reconceptualizing curricula offer nurse educators expanded and transcendent metaphors for reconceiving curricula and hold the promise of new, enlightened unions when, for nearly 25 years, the marriage of Tyler and nursing education has seemed immutable. Yet, we wonder how nursing faculty and students, other disciplines in higher education, and health care institutions will respond to curricula that speak of dialogue, meaning, self-reflection, intuition, and praxis when they are accustomed to curricula that speak of behavioral objectives, outcome criteria, subject matter, and evaluation tools. It is through the use of metaphors that we can facilitate common understandings and create a sense of community.

Metaphor is defined in *The Random House Dictionary for Writers and Readers* (Grambs, 1990) as the "figure of speech denoting implied comparison; an imaginative or analogous term used in place of a given word or concept, or an expressive and comparable figurative term" (p. 197). Eisner (1985) believes that "metaphor breaks the bonds of conventional usage to exploit the power of connotation and analogy. It capitalizes on surprise by putting meanings into new combinations and through such combinations awakens our senses" (p. 226).

Through the use of metaphors as a form of literary art, it may be possible for educators to do as Greene (1978) indicates: "to come in contact with ourselves, to recover a lost spontaneity" (p. 2). Ricoeur (1981) characterizes metaphor as an innovative linguistic method of discourse that has the potential to redescribe or represent reality. Metaphors allow a world of meaning to be disclosed rather than imposed (Ricoeur, 1981).

The use of metaphors establishes a forum for dialogue and promotes action toward change. Communication will be enhanced and relationships strengthened as the meanings of the curriculum revolution are shared with others in this way. We have discovered that the experiences of Alice and other characters in *Alice's Adventures in Wonderland* (Carroll, 1865) are not unlike the experiences of students of nursing. This paper presents *Alice in Wonderland* as a metaphor for sharing the lived experience of nursing education. We hope it discloses a world of meaning to you.

INTRODUCTION

On July 4, 1862 Charles Dodgson, a 30-year-old mathematical lecturer at Christ Church in Oxford, England, took the three small daughters of Dean Liddell on a boat ride. They had tea on the bank at Godstow and he told them the story of "Alice's Adventures Underground." He reportedly invented it as he went along. Later, Dodgson began to write the tales he had invented. He submitted the manuscript to the Claredon Press to print at his own expense and under the pen name of Lewis Carroll. The Claredon Press printed 2,000 copies in 1865.

The lived experience of Alice begins with she and her sister sitting under a tree on a quiet afternoon. Alice is bored. Suddenly, a white rabbit wearing a waistcoat and looking at a pocket watch runs close by her. He is saying to himself, "Oh, dear! Oh, dear! I shall be too late" (Carroll, p. 1).

Burning with curiosity, Alice starts to her feet, runs across the field, and down into a large rabbit hole after him, never considering how in the world she is to get out again. She finds herself falling, but she falls very slowly and has plenty of time to look about her and wonder what is going to happen next. Alice enters a world like no other she has ever experienced.

Alice finds a bottle on a glass table. It is labeled, "Drink me." Because it is not marked poison, Alice ventures to taste it, and finding it very nice ("it had, in fact, a sort of mixed flavor of cherry tart, custard, pineapple, roast turkey, toffy, and hot buttered toast" [p. 8]), she soon finishes drinking all of it. From that point on, her life becomes "curiouser and curiouser" (p. 11).

She grows large. She grows small. She experiences self-doubt, uncertainty, ignorance, and changing perspectives.

> Dear, dear! How queer everything is today! And yesterday things went on just as usual. I wonder if I've been changed in the night? Let me think: Was I the same when I got up this morning? I almost think I can remember feeling a little different. But if I'm not the same, the next question is, who in the world am I? Ah, that's the great puzzle. [p. 13]

The changes in her very being are complicated by the new acquaintances she makes in this new world: Humpty Dumpty, Caterpillar, Cheshire Cat, Mock Turtle, Gryphon, and the Queen.

So many out-of-the-way things have happened to Alice recently, that she begins to think that very few things indeed are really impossible. Alice has entered a land in which inconsistency and illogical events appear to be inevitable and so convincing.

We believe Alice's experiences to be similar to those of students entering the world of nursing education. Nursing school is also a world unlike any other. Life as a student of nursing can be very curious; students may experience a loss of identity, self-doubt, uncertainty, and radical changes of perspective. When Alice asks, "Do cats eat bats?" or "Do bats eat cats?" (p. 5), we can hear faculty asking "Does theory follow practice?" or "Does practice follow theory?" For, you see, (not unlike Alice) as we cannot answer convincingly either question, it does not matter which way we ask it.

ALICE'S EXPERIENCE WITH THE CATERPILLAR

Let us now assume that Alice has begun her experience as a nursing student. In Carroll's tale, there are two characters who are comparable to nursing educators.

The first is the Caterpillar, whom we liken to one of Alice's theory teachers. The Caterpillar plays a significant role in Alice's experiences in her new world. Unfortunately, he is a very controlling and paternalistic creature, just as are some nurse educators.

The Caterpillar, (i.e., nursing faculty member), asks Alice to repeat a poem. Alice folds her hands as if to gain some composure and begins to quote verbatim the didactic material that she has been "fed" by the theory teacher:

> You are old, Father William, the young man said,
>   And your hair has become very white;
> And yet you incessantly stand on your head—
>   Do you think, at your age, it is right? [p. 46]

Alice proceeds to recite this eight-paragraph poem very confidently. She feels very proud of her precise, entertaining recitation. The Caterpillar says nothing concerning the fact that Alice is able to quote the long, involved poem almost perfectly. Instead, he states that her recitation was not quite right.

How often do we as educators only point out that which a student has not done perfectly and concentrate all our comments on what is wrong with the assignment or performance? There is something positive that can be identified in most all assignments. We need not only point out all the negative things.

At this point in the story, Alice is only three inches tall. She indicates to the Caterpillar that she is not very happy about her size. She says, "Three inches is such a wretched height to be" (p. 47). This statement offends the Caterpillar who himself is only three inches tall. Alice has to defend her statement for fear of further irritating the creature. Quickly she points out that the problem with being three inches tall is just a problem for her because she is not used to it. Students are often very concerned that they not offend faculty. They are concerned that they may be graded or evaluated differently from classmates who have pleased the faculty member. Perhaps faculty should be as concerned with not offending students. Students are paying to learn. Are students' feelings not as important as those of faculty?

In Carroll's story the Caterpillar then crawls away and class is over. As he is leaving, almost as an afterthought, he says, "One side will make you grow taller, and the other side will make you grow shorter" (p. 48). Alice believes this is important information that she should know more about, owing to the fact that she is not happy with being three inches tall. She wonders to herself: "side of what?" (p. 48). The Caterpillar is completely out of sight before she can ask for clarification. The dialogue is over. How often do faculty expect students to perform and produce without giving them adequate information to meet expectations?

The Caterpillar exemplifies some negative aspects of professional nursing education: (1) the teacher's tendency to criticize students' work, rather than acknowledging positive accomplishments, (2) the importance placed on the educator's feelings and the lack of concern for the students' feelings, and (3) the teacher's inclination to withhold important information from students.

ALICE'S ENCOUNTER WITH THE CHESHIRE CAT

Alice's clinical instructor, the Cheshire Cat, is much like the Caterpillar in the manner in which it interacts with Alice. When Alice encounters the Cheshire Cat for the first time in the pre-clinical conference, it is grinning from ear to ear.

"Please would you tell me," says Alice, the student nurse, a little timidly (in her best student fashion), for she is not sure whether it is good manners for her to speak first, "why do you grin like that?"

"I'm a Cheshire Cat," says the instructor, "and that's *why!*" The last word is said with such violence that Alice jumps.

Eventually, she takes courage and speaks again: "I didn't know that Cheshire Cats always grinned; in fact, I didn't know that cats *could* grin at all." "We all can," says the Cat (instructor) "and most of us do" (p. 58).

Showing some assertiveness, Alice says politely, "I don't know of any that do" (p. 58). She is feeling quite good to have engaged the instructor in conversation.

Crushing any initiative for learning that poor Alice possesses, the Cheshire Cat replies, "You don't know much and that's a fact" (p. 58).

In spite of this encounter, Alice does not withdraw from the program, and the next morning, she encounters the instructor when she reports to the clinical area. The Cheshire Cat (instructor) only grins when it sees Alice. It *looks* good-natured enough, thinks Alice. Still, it has very long claws and a great many teeth, so she feels that it ought to be treated with great respect.

"Dr. Cheshire," she begins timidly, as she does not at all know whether it will like the name, however, the Cat only grins a little wider, "would you please tell me which way I ought to go from here?"

"That depends a good deal on where you want to get to," says the Cat (p. 63).

Alice, thinking of her many learning needs, says, "I don't much care where . . ." (p. 63).

The Cheshire Cat not permitting her to finish, interrupts saying, "Then it doesn't matter which way you go" (p. 63).

Alice mumbles, "so long as I get somewhere and graduate."

"Oh, you're sure to do that," says the Cat, "if you go the way I tell you to go" (p. 63).

Alice ponders this remark for a moment and then asks, "What sort of people are here?" (p. 64).

"Everyone here is mad," states the instructor, the Cat.

"But I don't want to go among mad people," says Alice (p. 64).

"Oh, you can't help that," says the instructor, "we're all mad here. I'm mad and you're mad" (p. 64).

"How do you know I'm mad?" asks Alice (p. 64).

"You must be," says the Cat, "or you wouldn't be here" (p. 64).

"How do you know that you are mad?" asks Alice (p. 64).

"Well, a dog's not mad," says the cat, "and it growls when it's angry and it wags its tail when it's pleased. I growl when I'm pleased and wag my tail when I'm angry. Therefore, I must be mad."

"I call it purring, not growling," says Alice (p. 64).

"Call it what you like," says the Cheshire Cat, "it's still growling."

This type of convoluted responding to questions is frequently encountered by students in their interactions with faculty. Double messages are sent, leaving the student to wonder about the meanings of the words and gestures of faculty.

Throughout this exchange, the Cheshire Cat continuously vanishes and reappears. Finally, Alice says, "I wish you wouldn't keep appearing and vanishing so suddenly; you make one quite giddy" (p. 66).

"All right," says the Cat, and this time it vanishes quite slowly, beginning with the end of the tail, and ending with the grin, which remains for some time after the rest of the Cat has gone.

Like the grin of the Cheshire Cat, the influence of the nurse educator on the student persists long after the pedagogic experience has ended.

ALICE'S EXPERIENCES WITH THE MOCK TURTLE AND THE GRYPHON

Alice's conversation with the Mock Turtle and the Gryphon can be likened to nursing students from different types of programs comparing their curricula and the faculty they have encountered. The exchange may also elucidate the lived experiences of nurses of different eras as they reflect on their adventures in nursing school.

The Mock Turtle said, "We had the best of educations—in fact, we went to school every day."

"I've been to day-school, too," said Alice, "you needn't be so proud as all that."

"With extras?" asked the Mock Turtle a little anxiously.

"Yes," replied Alice, "we learned French and music."

"And washing?" said the Mock Turtle.

"Certainly not!" said Alice indignantly.

"Ah! Then yours wasn't a really good school," said the Mock Turtle in a tone of great relief. "Now at ours they had at the end of the bill, 'French, music, and washing—extra.'"

"You couldn't have wanted it much," said Alice, "living at the bottom of the sea."

"I couldn't afford to learn it," said the Mock Turtle with a sigh. "I only took the regular course."

"What was that?" inquired Alice.

"Reeling and Writhing, of course, to begin with," the Mock Turtle replied; "and then the different branches of Arithmetic—Ambition, Distraction, Uglification, and Derision."

"I never heard of 'Uglification,'" Alice ventured to say.

"Well, then," said the Gryphon, "if you don't know what to uglify is, you *are* a simpleton."

Alice did not feel encouraged to ask any more questions about it, so she turned to the Mock Turtle, and said, "What else had you to learn?"

"Well, there was Mystery," the Mock Turtle replied, counting off the subjects on his flappers, "Mystery, ancient and modern, with Seaography; then Drawling—the Drawling master was an old conger eel, that used to come once a week; *he* taught us Drawling, Stretching, and Fainting in Coils."

"What was *that* like?" said Alice.

"Well, I can't show it to you, myself," the Mock Turtle replied; "I'm too stiff. And the Gryphon never learned it."

"Hadn't time," said the Gryphon; "I went to the Classical Master, though. He was on old crab, *he* was."

"I never went to him," the Mock Turtle responded with a sigh; "he taught Laughing and Grief, they used to say."

"And how many hours a day did you do lessons?" said Alice.

"Ten hours the first day," said the Mock Turtle, "nine the next, and so on."

"What a curious plan!" exclaimed Alice.

"That's the reason they're called lessons," the Gryphon remarked, "because they lessen from day to day." [Carroll, pp. 102–104]

ALICE AND HUMPTY DUMPTY

As Alice, the student, continues her educational journey through the looking glass, she comes upon a curious-looking egg. As she comes closer, the egg becomes larger and larger, and more familiar. When she comes within a few yards of it, she sees that it has eyes, a nose, and a mouth; and, when she comes very close to it, she sees clearly that it is—can it be? It is—Humpty Dumpty— the traditional, objective and content-driven curriculum himself!

There he is, in all his glory, sitting with his legs crossed like a Turk, on top of a high, narrow wall. The wall is so narrow that Alice wonders how Humpty Dumpty can keep his balance.

As Alice begins to interact and speak with Humpty Dumpty, the curriculum, it immediately becomes obvious that there is an uncomfortable tension between the two of them. Alice questions why Humpty Dumpty, the curriculum, is resting on such a perilous foundation: "That wall is very narrow!" Alice exclaims. "Wouldn't you feel safer here on the ground—that is, closer to the real world?"

Humpty Dumpty, the curriculum, growls out: "Of course I won't fall—why, there's no chance of it. But, if I did fall, the King of Behaviorist Objectives has promised me—with his very own mouth—to send all of his horses and all of his men—the whole Tylerian Brigade. They would pick me up in a minute and we would start afresh all over again!"

Why, Alice thinks, he talks about it just as if it were a game!

Alice and Humpty Dumpty, the curriculum, continue playing the verbal debate game, each one taking turns in choosing the subjects (of papers), the coursework, and the programs.

The dialogue, however, is egocentric and superficial. Humpty Dumpty and Alice quarrel continuously over knowledge, facts, truth, meaning, and reality.

The dialogue continues. Neither Humpty Dumpty nor Alice attempt to view the world through the eyes of the other—neither tries to bridge the gap that exists from the top of the high, narrow curriculum wall, to the soft, green earth of the real world below.

Finally, in exasperation, Alice challenges Humpty Dumpty by saying: "There is no meaning. Come off that wall and walk this ground with me."

Humpty Dumpty is startled and responds sharply: "If you could *see* whether I'm singing or not, you've sharper eyes than most!" (p. 233).

Alice falls silent—her voice is lost.

There is a long pause. Finally, Alice timidly asks: "Is that all?" (p. 235).

"That's all," snaps Humpty Dumpty. "Goodby" (p. 235).

That was rather sudden, thinks Alice, but, after such a very strong hint that she ought to be going, she feels that it would hardly be civil to stay. So, she gets up and holds out her hand. "Goodbye until we meet again," she says as cheerfully as she can.

Humpty Dumpty replies: "I shouldn't know you again if we ever did meet. You're so exactly like all other students—your face is just the same as everyone's—two eyes, a nose in the middle, mouth under . . . ."

As he never opens his eyes or takes any further notice of her, Alice says "Goodbye" once more, and, as she graduates from school, she can't help murmuring to herself as she receives her degree: "Well, of all the unsatisfactory experiences I ever had. . . ."

She never finishes her sentence, for at that moment, a heavy crash shakes the earth from end to end.

To paraphrase Jean Watson's (1988) argument for a curriculum revolution:

> In so deciding of the need for curriculum change, the school is publicly acknowledging that Humpty Dumpty has fallen, and the pieces cannot be put back together again. We believe that today the profession of nursing is being challenged to create a new, professional nurse, who is a full health and human caring professional, or else become obsolete.

ALICE IN THE QUEEN'S COURT

Alice's final experience in Wonderland occurs in the Queen's court. This portion of our metaphor provides symbolic representation of the curriculum revolution. This is our interpretation of the events at court. "The Queen of Accreditation!" "The Queen of Accreditation!" Into the courtroom enters a full procession complete with soldiers and last of all—the Queen of Accreditation!

The Queen of Accreditation points to the faculty of the schools of nursing who are all working furiously to make the curriculum look just right and to meet the explicit guidelines of what constitutes a curriculum.

"What are they doing?" asks the Queen of Accreditation.

"May it please your majesty," says a lowly faculty member, "we are trying. . . ."

"I see," says the Queen of Accreditation. "Off with their accreditation!"

The Queen has only one way of settling all difficulties whether they be great or small—off with their accreditation!

The Queen is seated on her throne and a great crowd assembles around her.

The Judge is the King of Accreditation. There is a jury, too, made of 12 Board of Review members.

Standing in chains before all of them is the faculty of the Revolutionary School of Nursing.

"Read the accusation!" exclaims the Judge. On this command, the White Rabbit unrolls a scroll and reads as follows: "The Queen of Accreditation, she made some rules—all on a summer day; the Revolutionary School of Nursing, they stole the rules, and took them all away."

"Consider the verdict," the Judge says to the jury.

"No, not yet!" says the White Rabbit. "There's a great deal more to come before that."

Alice, the nursing student, is called to the witness stand.

"What do you know of this business?" the Judge asks Alice.

"I have learned to know myself, to question, and to practice nursing in creative ways," responds Alice. Alice feels proud that she is able to think critically and innovatively for she is indeed a student in the Revolutionary School of Nursing.

The Judge reads from his book: "Rule 4-2 says that all persons who question and who exhibit independence and creativity must leave the court at once."

"That's not a rule," says Alice, "you've just invented it."

"It's the oldest rule in the book," replies the Judge, "besides, we have always done it that way!"

"There's more evidence," says the White Rabbit, holding up an envelope.

"What's in it?" asks the Queen of Accreditation.

The Rabbit says: "I haven't opened it, but it seems to be an essay examination written by Alice, the student, and given to a faculty member to be graded."

The White Rabbit opens it and exclaims: "It isn't an essay exam after all, it is a self-reflective journal!"

"That proves the guilt, of course!" says the Queen of Accreditation.

"Let the jury consider the verdict," says the Judge.

"No, No," responds the Queen of Accreditation, "sentence first—verdict afterwards."

"That is nonsense," Alice says loudly.

"Off with their accreditation!" the Queen shouts.

Many more characters from *Alice in Wonderland* could be used as metaphors to explore the lived experiences of students in nursing school. We hope our use of metaphor has transcended some of the limitations and restrictions of our everyday language and allowed a different view to be disclosed.

REFERENCES

Carroll, L. (1865). *Alice's adventures in wonderland.* Oxford, England: Claredon Press.

Eisner, E. W. (1985). *The educational imagination: On the design and evaluation of school programs.* New York: Macmillan.

Grambs, D. (Ed.). (1990). *The Random house dictionary for writers and readers.* New York: Random House.

Greene, M. (1978). *Landscapes of learning.* New York: Teacher's College Press.

Ricoeur, P. (1981). *Hermeneutics and the human sciences.* New York: Cambridge University Press.

Watson, J. (1988). Human caring as moral context for nursing education. *Nursing and Health Care, 9,* 423–425.

6

A Community-Based
Primary Health Care Program
for Integration of Research, Practice,
and Education

Beverly J. McElmurry,
Susan M. Swider, and Kathleen Norr

This chapter describes a demonstration program which has been developing at the University of Illinois at Chicago over the past ten years. This program focuses on the development of a university setting that is responsive to the primary health care concerns of an urban population, and that uses the project staff's expertise in women's health research and education to inform our understanding of women's health problems and their resolution. Key elements underlying this program that can be viewed as global concerns in health care are:

The project described in this chapter is partially supported by the W. K. Kellogg Foundation, the Robert R. McCormick Charitable Trust, the Chicago Community Trust, the U. S. Office of Minority Health, and the University of Illinois at Chicago.

1. recognition of women as key persons to target in facilitation of health promotion and maintenance for families and communities;

2. acceptance of primary health care (PHC) as a global strategy for focusing attention on the minimum essential health care needs of people in areas such as nutrition, prevention of communicable diseases, housing, and safety;

3. recognition of the interaction between health and social conditions and the importance of self-care and community competency in maintaining basic health and health care services; and

4. continued search for the means to develop health professional and community member collaboration at the grass-roots level to define health problems and work toward their resolution.

This program is implemented through a model that links professional health research, service, and education in health care provided to the community. Linking these activities enriches and strengthens all three areas. The maintenance of ongoing community-based service projects provides a testing ground for new knowledge; the integration of research findings into health service delivery improves the quality of health care services; and the opportunity for students to relate the didactic content of their courses to ongoing programs of service and research provides an education that is relevant to urban health concerns and incorporates the primary health care approach.

BACKGROUND

The project staff members (nurses, advocates, and others) like to depict the Primary Health Care in Urban Communities project through the use of overlapping circles (Figure 6–1). This basic diagram can be used to illustrate the various locations of activities such as provision of a parent support network, establishment of a teen center, or provision of peer support education for the prevention of AIDS.

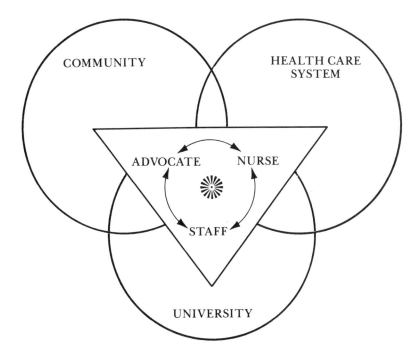

Figure 6–1
Locations for Nurse Advocate Team Activities

This figure also illustrates the importance of a community-based demonstration program, i.e., it provides a means for integrating research, education, and practice. This figure is embedded in the context of PHC, with particular concern for essential or basic health care for all people. This implementation of PHC emphasizes community-focused care, promoting and maintaining health, interaction of health with the development of self-reliant communities, and nurse and community partnerships in health care.

Note that the term "primary health care" is different from "primary care." We, the project staff members, use the term PHC to capture the idea of ensuring access to essential health care for all residents of a community. This is care which is provided at a level that the community can afford and in a manner which solicits the full participation of community members. In PHC, the definition of health is broad and fosters a health and development perspective. At Alma Ata, the World Health Organization (WHO) defined PHC in the following way.

> [PHC is] Essential health care based on practical, scientifically sound and socially acceptable methods and technology made universally accessible to individuals and their families in the community through their full participation and at a cost that the community and country can afford to maintain at every stage of their development in the spirit of self-reliance and self-determination. It forms an integral part both of the country's health system, of which it is the central function and focus, and of the overall social and economic development of the community. It is the first level of contact of individuals, the family and community with the national health system bringing health care as close as possible to where people live and work, and constitutes the first element of a continuing health care process. [WHO, 1978, p. 3]

We have tried to apply this definition of PHC in Chicago by asking ourselves: what can inner city residents do as individuals and as a community to improve their health, and what can we do to facilitate the improvement of their health? Such questions evolved from our experience with low income inner city women and their children (McElmurry, et al., 1987; Swider & McElmurry, 1990; McElmurry, et al., 1990). Many of the women we had worked with prior to the implementation of the project were unable to obtain quality health care services responsive to their situations and sensitive to their ethnic and/or racial backgrounds. In our current demonstration program, we realize that the small teams we have in a variety of settings are not going to bring about the changes needed in American health care. However, we do think we are learning something which others will find useful and which will give voice to the health concerns of inner city women and their families.

ASPECTS OF THE DEMONSTRATION PROJECT

The inner city, with its violence and crime, is a tough place to live or work. Yet, if our key concern is primary health care, then it is necessary to find a way to strengthen grass-roots involvement in determining how to improve the health of the people in this community. A grass-roots group has several characteristics: "the capacities to tap local knowledge and resources; to respond to problems rapidly and creatively; and to maintain the flexibility needed in changing circumstances (Durning, 1989, pp. 6–7).

Our model of PHC has evolved over time and within the context of our situation. Our first task was to select a target community for the location of team activities. The definition of community can be quite varied. The key idea used by the project staff to define community is Grace's (1990) point that it is necessary to find the common shared interest that unites people in coordinated action. Examples of community as used in our program have incuded urban community areas, elementary schools, community-based health care settings, youth centers, and hospital maternity units.

Once the community is selected, community residents are recruited for training to become community health workers who will work in a team with community health nurses. Over the years, we have compiled a curriculum guide for the training of advocates, which is useful to trainees and the faculty and community agencies or members who help us with the training program. (An extensive discussion of the community health worker preparation can be found in Swider & McElmurry, 1990.)

Upon initiation of the training program, the nurse/advocate teams are asked to conduct community assessments. As they conduct the assessment of communities, there are several key questions asked:

- What are the essential health (broadly defined) concerns expressed by residents of this community?
- How important are the identified health concerns to community residents given the other community concerns or issues which they identify?

- Are there existing approaches or resources available to meet the health concerns expressed by community residents? For example, are there existing activities designed to teach community people to meet health needs via their own actions in order to foster self-reliance?

- Are the community residents aware of, supportive of, and involved with the existing approaches or resources designed to resolve health problems or concerns?

- Are the existing community approaches or resources for health designed to promote equity?

- Are the existing approaches to health concerns acceptable and affordable given the resources and social and economic conditions of the community?

- Are a variety of sectors of society involved in designing and implementing existing approaches to health concerns and promoting and maintaining the health of the community?

- Does the educational system for health professionals teach and promote research consistent with the health concerns of the community?

- Does the local government have structures to promote PHC services which include ongoing public debate about health needs and services in the context of the local culture and resources?

As noted earlier, over time, the PHC program has used various definitions of community. Regardless of location, however, the program has some key features in its structure or program components.

Although the overall project is housed in a university setting, the nurse/advocate teams work in community-based locations. The community locations for which advocates have been trained include the following examples:

- In an Hispanic community, the team is found in a comprehensive, free-standing, private clinic. In the black community, the team is located in a church basement.

- In the public education system, the team is found in schools, two that are primarily Hispanic and two that are mainly black.

Each school has a nurse and two advocates. The school compo-nent has been a recent evolvement (McElmurry & Newcomb, 1990).

- In another case, advocates have been prepared to work in an Hispanic community where the team will be housed in a multi-purpose youth center.

- In a hospital-based service project centered in the maternity unit, nurse/advocate teams provide health promotion and home visits to pregnant women and to new mothers and infants in selected low-income communities with high infant mortality rates (Barnes-Boyd, 1990).

PROJECT SUPPORT ACTIVITIES

The project's infrastructure or support activities are evolving and reflect our understanding of what is required to conduct a community-based demonstration project and to garner the neces-sary resources. Support activities include the establishment of the community data base, evaluation team, social policy analyst, peer support groups, and leadership development activities.

Community Data Base

To date, the community data base has been described in speeches at professional meetings (Montgomery, et al., 1989) and in print-outs provided to various community agencies. The organizing for-mat for the data base are the community areas. The data included are both the traditional health data and other data that are of spe-cial concern to urban health initiatives. Thus, the data cover gen-eral demographics, labor force characteristics, live births, infant deaths, deaths, public safety, and social control (A. Montgomery, personal communication, February 1991).

There are various uses for the community data which have been compiled. We have noted that when the health advocates present the data to members of their own community, they take time to think about the meaning of the data. Knowing that there are a number of health concerns in one's own community is different from presenting those concerns in the form of data which must be interpreted to one's neighbors. At times, the advocates have expressed their sense of the gloom the statistics convey. Their concern has been to balance the reality of the situation with the provision of hope or a "can do" approach to the development of community health services. They give serious thought to statistics which indicate that of the 1,308 births (1987) in their community, 66 percent were to mothers age 19 or younger, and 46 percent had eight or fewer years of education. Or, that out of a total population of 53,741, there were 22,178 recipients of Aid to Families With Dependent Children.

Evaluation Team

Aspects of evaluation have been a component of most of the grants obtained for the implementation of the PHC initiatives. The evaluation team has examined a variety of options for evaluation methods and foci. For the most part, the evaluation could be characterized as a multimethod and multimeasure approach in which we try to better understand the meaning of participatory evaluation. In this case, participatory evaluation as described by Feuerstein (1986) means that the measures make sense to health professionals as well as the community members whose help is needed to collect the data.

An example is the encounter form that advocates utilize to capture the essence of their service. It is a user-friendly form in that the advocates are able to record their work, and the evaluation team can later enter the data coded on the form directly into the computer.

We have learned to clearly differentiate evaluation activities which help us better understand the project and its effects or evolvement from those which focus on evaluation of individual performance. Over time, the advocates have found it helpful to obtain participant feedback on the usefulness of their presentations to the community.

Social Policy Analyst

A focus on grass-roots social policy development emerged sometime after implementation of the community-based nurse/advocate teams, as the staff became more aware that our usual way of examining health policy was professionally driven. Outside of the traditional community development literature, there was little guidance on how to develop a grass-roots social policy thrust in low income urban communities. Subsequently, a person with a social policy background was added to the project staff (McElmurry & Swider, 1987 to date) and asked to help the nurse/advocate teams identify a focus for grass-roots policy development. Eventually, all involved in the project agreed on the seriousness of violence as a public health concern in the inner city communities. Through focused discussion groups, the Hispanic community selected violence against women as an area of focus, and the black community selected the preservation of youth as a focus. The role of the social policy analyst was to help the community members define what they could do in response to the selected problem area and to make professional expertise available to them. In each case, the problem of violence has been addressed from a "positive" perspective, e.g., what can women do to recognize abuse and develop means for dealing with it, or how can we develop a youth center which incorporates a health component.

Over time, the social policy analyst became interested in the health concerns facing minority males. The project personnel recognized that this was a major urban problem, but there were only rare instances when multidisciplinary health groups met together with low income parents and their children to talk about what worked to keep young, urban males healthy. It has been decided that the initial effort will be to organize a conference in which community parents and their sons will meet with health professionals to share ideas on what has worked and what they would like to see as the future health agenda for urban males. It is our hope that this effort will become a coalition of family members, minority males, and health professionals who will continue to work together on shared health concerns.

Peer Support Groups

A component of the original training program for health advocates was the time set aside for them to meet as a group with the clinical psychologist on the project staff. These sessions were designed to focus on learning to identify feelings and develop problem-solving skills. Over time, the project staff members have recognized that peer support sessions are appropriate for professional personnel as well as for the community workers. The nurses need time to share their experiences and what they have learned about their role, and the staff members at the university need time to share what they are learning. For professionals, PHC as used in this demonstration, has led to reflection about shared decision making and negotiation with community residents. For example, the professionals have many opportunities to wrestle with questions or issues such as whether or when activities are professional perogatives or shared decisions.

Leadership Development Activities

A recent addition to the University's PHC activities has been the attainment of funding for a leadership development training program in which curricula for community leaders and health professionals will be developed (McElmurry & Sajid, 1990). This program is a joint effort of nursing and medicine to design a leadership training program in which experiential activities in the community are provided for both professionals and lay leaders. Selected community sites are designated as partners with the university in advancing knowledge about community-based health services.

FUTURE CHALLENGES

It is evident that there are many challenges facing the project personnel at this time. For example:

1. Is it possible to institutionalize a grass-roots, negotiated process approach to cooperative health initiatives by health professionals and community residents?

2. Can a PHC emphasis in community-based settings be sustained? The Canadian Public Health Association (1990) has used the term "sustainable development" to mean "the development of health programs that meet the needs of the present without compromising the ability of future generations to meet their own needs" (p. 5). Are we ready to establish national policies which lead to funding and other supports to sustain this focus?

3. Can the community health worker and nursing roles in community-based care be described in a manner that captures the skills needed for these roles and that wins the support of the community and nursing establishments?

4. Will the use and methods of participatory evaluation achieve agreement from both the community residents and the health professionals?

CONCLUSION

The demonstration project began with the following goals:

- Within the urban context or environment, university and community participants will implement PHC programs using a collaborative decision-making process.

- Given the structure of internal/external organizations, the collaborative decision-making program in PHC will maximize opportunities for community residents and health professionals to use their knowledge in advancing the health of people in targeted community areas.

- A collaborative decision-making program in PHC will function to increase the competency of community areas in addressing identified health and social problems. (This desired outcome captures empowerment in the sense used by Wheeler & Chinn [1989] of strength or solidarity in moving toward goals.)

- A sense of integrity (linkage) is achieved when the concepts of PHC and community empowerment are incorporated or adopted in other health policies and programs.

Developing a community-based nursing practice which integrates the traditional university functions of research, service, and education is consistent with the WHO resolution (1984) on the role of universities in contributing to human development and social justice. In particular, the point emphasized is that university personnel place themselves at the disposal of communities to the maximum of their capacity for the promotion of health and the provision of health care.

Nursing literature stresses the role of researchers in acute care clinical settings (Schulzenhofer, 1991; Knafl et al., 1987; McBride, et al., 1970), of establishing research programs in acute care settings (Hinshaw & Smeltzer, 1987; Chance & Hinshaw, 1980; Egan, McElmurry, & Jameson, 1981), and of the value of collaboration between education and service settings (Walker, 1985; Barrell & Hamric, 1986; Clark, 1986). We find little literature, however, to guide us in establishing integrated (research, service, and education) services in low income urban settings. This is a curious situation as we face the future and the much touted movement from acute care settings to home care and community-based services. Yet, such integration services and demonstration models are imperative to the achievement of our educational goals. Can students appreciate the need for change in health care if we do not provide experiential opportunities for them to grabble with the issues?

REFERENCES

Barnes-Boyd, C. (1990 to date). *Reach futures.* A service project funded by the Healthy Tomorrows Partnership for Children Program, a collaborative program of the Office of Maternal and Child Health (USPHS) and the American Academy of Pediatrics (MCHIP grant) (MCJ 178507).

Barrell, L. M., & Hamric, A. B. (1986). Education and service: A collaborative model to improve patient care. *Nursing and Health Care, 7,* 497–503.

Canadian Public Health Association. (1990). *CPHA Position Paper 1 on sustainability and equity: Primary health care in developing countries.* Canada: Author.

Chance, H. C., & Hinshaw, A. S. (1980). Strategies for initiating a research program. *Journal of Nursing Administration, 10*(3), 32–39.

Clark, M. D. (1986). Unifying nursing. *Nursing Success Today, 3,* 10–14.

Diamond, S. (1990 to date). *Healthy sons, healthy families* conference. University of Chicago, Chicago, IL. U. S. Office of Minority Health.

Durning, A. B. (1989). Action at the grass–roots: Fighting poverty and environmental decline. *Worldwatch Paper 88.* Washington, DC: Worldwatch Institute.

Egan, E., McElmurry, B. J., & Jameson, H. M. (1981). Practice based research: Assessing your department's readiness. *Journal of Nursing Administration, 11,* 26–32.

Feuerstein, M. T. (1986). Evaluation development and community programmes with participants. *Partners in Evaluation.* London: Macmillan.

Grace, H. K. (1990). Building community: A conceptual perspective. *International Journal of W. K. Kellogg Foundation, 1*(1), 20–22.

Hinshaw, A. S., & Smeltzer, C. H. (1987). Research challenges and programs for practice settings. *Journal of Nursing Administration, 17*(7 & 8), 20–26.

Knafl, K. A., Hagle, M. E., Bevis, M. E., & Kirchhoff, K. T. (1987). Clinical nurse researchers: Strategies for success. *Journal of Nursing Administration, 17*(10), 27–31.

McBride, M. A., Diers, D., & Schmidt, R. L. (1970). The nurse-researcher: The crucial hyphen. *American Journal of Nursing, 70*(6), 1256–1260.

McElmurry, B. J., & Newcomb, J. N. (1990). *PHC for urban school children.* The Partners in Health component of the Nation of Tomorrow Project, funded by the University of Illinois at Chicago, 1990 to 1994.

McElmurry, B. J., & Sajid, A. W. (1990 to date). *Leadership for PHC: Partnerships between the community and university.* W. K. Kellogg Foundation (S. M. Poslusny, Project Director).

McElmurry, B. J., & Swider, S. M. (1987 to date). *Collaborative decision making: Community health workers and health care professionals* (W. K. Kellogg Foundation); PHC in urban communities: Social policy component (with S. Diamond, Robert R. McCormick Charitable Foundation); and preparation of lay health advocates in Chicago community areas (Chicago Community Trust).

McElmurry, B. J., Swider, S. M., Bless, C., Murphy, D., Montgomery, A., Norr, K., Irvin, Y., Gantes, M., & Fisher, M. (1990). Community health advocacy: Primary health care nurse/advocate teams in urban communities. In NLN *Perspectives in Nursing 1989–1991.* New York: National League for Nursing.

McElmurry, B. J., Swider, S. M., Grimes, M., Dan, A., Irvin, Y., & Lourenco, S. V. (1987). Health advocacy for young, low income inner city women. *Advances in Nursing Science, 9*(9), 62–75.

Montgomery, A., Fisher, M., Sullivan, J., McElmurry, B. J., & Swider, S. M. (1989). *A computerized database in primary health care: An application of the community diagnosis laboratory.* Unpublished paper. American Public Health Association, Chicago, IL.

Schulzenhofer, K. K. (1991). Scholarly pursuit in the clinical setting: An obligation of professional nursing. *Journal of Professional Nursing, 7*(1), 10–15.

Swider, S. M., & McElmurry, B. J. (1990). A women's health perspective in primary health care: A nursing and community health worker demonstration project in urban America. *Family and Community Health, 13*(3), 1–17.

Walker, D. D. (1985). Nursing education and service: The payoffs of partnerships. *Nursing and Health Care, 6,* 189–191.

Wheeler, C. E., & Chinn, P. L. (1989). *Peace & Power: A Handbook of Feminist Process* (2nd ed.). New York: National League for Nursing.

World Health Organization. (1984). *The role of universities in the strategies of health for all: A contribution to human development and social justice.* Resolution adopted by the 37th World Health Assembly (Resolution WHA 37.31). Geneva: Author.

World Health Organization. (1978). *Primary health care: Alma Ata Conference.* Geneva: Author.

7

An Interdisciplinary Clinical Practicum: The Demise of a Successful Community Project

Julia C. Tiffany

In setting the tone and direction for this year's conference, "Community Building and Activism," Patty Hawken (1990), President of the National League for Nursing, urges nurses to "respond to the challenge to reclaim our communities" (p. B). She describes the theme as representing "a new momentum aimed at mobilizing the nursing community's strength, expertise, compassion and vision to create a new brand of health care delivery" (p. B). Her message inspired my return to and reflection on the interdisciplinary clinical practicum that involved my energies, resources, fascination, and commitment for four years. It would have been easier and more personally comfortable to share this project as a shining example of one way to create new possibilities in service and education. The project, however, has ended. This paper, therefore, explores the problems we encountered and analyzes the forces that led to the demise of the Interdisciplinary Project (IDP). Through our experience, perhaps others too will learn.

BIRTH OF THE INTERDISCIPLINARY PROJECT

The IDP, launched in 1980, linked social welfare, medical, and nursing students in a community-based interdisciplinary clinical practicum. The project created a unique learning environment for students and vital linkages between an underserved frail elderly population and community resources. Students, residents, building managers, program administrators, and service providers considered the project valuable and vital. It served as a model for the development of other interdisciplinary projects. With such success, what then led to its demise? The answers to that question lie embedded in the project's structure and evolution.

In 1980, the nursing director of a local community health agency experienced increasing frustration at her agency's lack of resources and ability to meet basic health and social welfare needs of frail elderly people, particularly those living in the inner city. She called together deans and directors from local nursing, medical, and social welfare programs to explore the problem. This group's early discussions focused on the unmet needs of the elderly. They explored ways to collaborate and to advocate for resources. Gradually, however, their vision and definition of the problem and its resolution possibilities broadened and deepened. They began to fantasize and to link the learning needs of students with the health and social needs of this population.

An idea took form. The group envisioned a practicum where students could learn together—a setting where they could experience one another's roles and theoretical mind-sets, a place where they would work collaboratively to identify and meet the needs of this underserved population. The interdisciplinary project was born from their creativity, their collaboration, and their willingness to risk trying something new. It was also born of their abilities to convey their vision and fire the enthusiasm and commitment of others. Each administrator recruited personnel from his or her own department or school and committed resources to the project. Faculty members with collective expertise in gerontology and community health care were joined by a nurse from the community health agency who had been serving this urban elderly population. The group members came to see themselves and to be known as the IDP faculty, regardless of their prior role definitions.

As faculty came together, a crisis was building for a group of elderly residents living in a dilapidated urban hotel. The building, recently purchased by a conglomerate interested in major renovations, was being torn apart even as managers and local agencies worked desperately to relocate residents. The faculty team selected this building and its residents as the site for the first interdisciplinary experience.

Given the context of a pending crisis, the first teams of students quickly became involved not only with assessment but also with actively meeting needs and advocating for residents with city authorities and other health and social providers. They found themselves exposed to individual health and social problems facing each resident, and also to the political, economic, and environmental forces impinging on these people as a group. A sense of urgency engendered by the demolition of the hotel and the need to relocate residents, most of whom were moving to a nearby congregate housing unit still under construction, facilitated a sense of camaraderie and interdependence among the students as well as with the faculty, residents, and the management of the new building. Fournier and Stedman (1982), two of the faculty working on the project during this initial phase, graphically illustrate the significance and depth of learning experienced by students as they worked with residents to meet and resolve the crisis.

> Locating students in a social system experiencing crisis proved to be a key element in promoting heightened learning with respect to role-blurring; interdisciplinary and interagency teamwork; community assessment; profound contrasts between professional, municipal, and capitalist responses to human need; and extremely disciplined utilization of the press to bring pressure upon local officials. [p. 10]

In 1982, three of the project's four original faculty members, within months of one another, chose to leave for personal reasons. None of the reasons included dissatisfaction with the project. In each case, new members were recruited by the person leaving. I was one of them. The remaining faculty member, a social worker, introduced us to the workings of the project. His enthusiasm and clarity of mission and process proved contagious. The new team adopted the framework and methods used by previous faculty without question.

In the same two years, all of the original administrators whose vision had created the project, had also moved on. Only in hindsight did the significance of these dual events emerge. At the time, however, the project continued without pause.

By 1982, tenants from the hotel were well settled in their new apartments. A resident council, generated with the assistance of student participation, actively engaged in social and governing activities. Students began to approach inhabitants living in a neighboring building to assess their individual and group needs.

THE PROJECT IN ACTION

The group dynamics and students' routines proved fascinating. First-year medical students, with four clinical hours a week and a focus on learning to communicate and utilize beginning assessment skills, joined junior social welfare students whose 16 practice hours a week focused on assessing social needs and interfacing with established community resources and agencies. Senior nursing students with eight clinical hours a week focused both on assessing health needs and interfacing with other resources. Three to five students constituted each interdisciplinary team. Teams, assigned to geographic areas in each of the two, and later four, buildings, were responsible for case-finding and resident contact as well as for follow-up with residents identified by prior students.

Early in the morning of each joint clinical day, students and faculty met in a large group to discuss student experiences, concerns, and questions. At times the group focused on didactic content, or media presentations specific to the elderly or to working in the community. Following the group meeting, teams met to determine their plan for the day before dispersing to work individually or in groups.

Students visited previously identified clients who evidenced a variety of health and social problems. Difficulties with daily activities such as shopping, transportation to appointments, personal care, and home management proved common. Total lack of medical care for some residents was juxtaposed with others who had several physicians involved simultaneously. Social isolation, loneliness, depression, physical infirmities, and fears of being accosted in an area frequented by prostitutes, drug addicts, and vagrants generated a variety of problems.

Students quickly learned to identify available resources in the community. They practiced networking and advocacy to link residents with needed services. The community health nurse's involvement on the project proved vital here with her knowledge of, and contacts with, community resources and agencies.

At times, students worked through resident groups to create needed resources. Providing craft and exercise classes, establishing routine shopping runs through a regional transportation service, inviting students from a local hairdressing school to provide services, and negotiating with the city's public works department to clear nearby brick sidewalks of ice and to install a handrail to make walking safer, were but a few of the interventions they made.

Students reached out beyond the defined population of clients identified by prior project participants. They talked with building managers and staff. They knocked on doors to introduce themselves and the services available through the project. Most residents, eager for company and the opportunity to relate their needs and stories, readily invited them in. Frequently, residents recommended that students visit friends or neighbors they saw as having problems or needing help.

Because of the erratic and part-time nature of their availability, their frequent turnover, and their focus on learning, faculty discouraged students from fostering dependency by meeting clients' needs directly. Rather, they encouraged students to seek more permanent resources and solutions and to work toward termination from the time of initial contact. This proved difficult for students and residents alike. It seemed so much easier to "just go and do that little bit of shopping" rather than enter the lengthy and, at times, frustrating process of connecting clients with health or social services so that shopping could be done on a continuing basis.

STUDENT RESPONSES TO THE PROJECT

With faculty support and intervention, most students gradually defined roles for themselves individually and within teams. Students witnessed faculty working collaboratively in the context of large group meetings and through home visits with students. They became more comfortable with role blurring and using one another as resources. Fournier and Stedman (1982) describe their learning and responses.

> By testing out where their own discipline overlapped or was similar to others, students demonstrated growth with respect to conceptualizing the parameters of their own disciplines. They didn't always think alike or approach problems similarly, but most developed a strong commitment to the real need to act together and use each other appropriately. [p. 11]

Anxious at first and resistant to the lack of structure, ambiguity of task, unclarity of role, and need for self-motivation in the context of working in teams, most students, in the course of their time in the project, became excited and wonderfully creative—at least, and perceived only in hindsight, the nursing and social welfare students did.

The majority of first-year medical students experienced and exhibited even more frustration and bewilderment on joining the project than their counterparts. New to the study of medicine and eager for the thrill and challenge of early clinical experiences, these students chaffed as they encountered peers assigned to hospitals and clinics with *real* doctors. At the instigation of the medical students and also in response to resident needs, one and then two screening clinics were added to the semester's experience, providing needed structure and focus for all students. This created a learning context seen as more reflective of and appropriate to the physician's traditional role.

The project's lack of formal structure and expectation for creating new models of service delivery in an interdisciplinary and community context required at least a beginning sense of professional self and professional role. In hindsight, it becomes clear that this expectation and environment were inappropriate for first-year students of any kind. Why did this insight not occur to us at the time? Perhaps our commitment to the ideals of the project and our attention, which focused introspectively on the learning of students and the immediate needs of clients, blinded us to, what seems now, a glaringly evident observation. One lesson in planning such a project in the future requires careful attention to the level of student, the mix of students, and the appropriateness of the learning experience.

THE BEGINNING OF THE END

In 1984, the medical faculty member left. The project format and process shifted though its goals remained the same. Finding no one willing to replace him, the physician recommended that medical student assignment to the project be left to the health educator responsible for student placements. The educator, though acknowledging the project's worth, believed strongly that it was not an appropriate experience for first-year medical students—at least not for a full semester. She negotiated three-week rotations for medical students each semester during which time they would be integrated into existing teams and supervised on-site by nursing and social welfare faculty. Their primary role and learning, however, was to be centered around the screening clinics. Not wanting to lose the important experiences gleaned from work with medical students, we agreed to this new arrangement.

Although valuable learning and interventions continued to occur, the content and character of the project changed. In hindsight, our investment in maintaining the project as a three-way interdisciplinary experience resulted in our replicating traditional professional roles with medical students dropping in, focusing on physical assessment, performing perfunctory follow-up, then leaving. Nursing and social welfare students and faculty remained to create and maintain the ongoing structure, character, focus, and work of the project. The very core of the interdisciplinary project which called for a re-creation and redefinition of professional roles and relationships was breaking down or, at least, dramatically changing—and all without our conscious awareness.

The physician's departure was followed by the semiretirement of the social welfare faculty member one year later. He also failed to find a replacement, at least one willing to perform in other than a perfunctory and part-time basis during the semester he was not teaching. The disciplines of medicine and social welfare are not attuned to direct student teaching in the field. Rather, both depend on agency staff and practitioners to serve as preceptors with responsibility for creating students' learning environments and experiences. The fact that two physicians and one social worker broke ranks and worked personally with students in the field proved an anomaly. They came early in the project when the adrenaline surge of creativity remained high. Finding replacements during a time of maintenance proved harder to achieve. At the time, I understood the significance of the social worker's leaving solely within this context. It is only now, through the passage of time and insight gleaned from reflection, that I truly understand the significance of this man's leaving. Retrospection and distance often generate clarity in this way.

The project had survived and thrived because of the dedication, tenacity, and teamwork of faculty and students involved over the years. The original excitement in and commitment to creating something new and unique, working collaboratively, and serving a population so in need survived even through major changes of personnel. One force, however, had held constant during all that time—the presence and influence of a dynamic and knowledgeable social worker who had been with the project from the beginning. Because we worked collaboratively and as peers without the formality of a hierarchical structure, his influence was covert. Nevertheless, his senior status, force of personality, and professional experience and competence made him a strong leader and driving force in the project. His departure created a chasm that could not be bridged, particularly since we were not consciously aware of this event's impact and repercussions.

During the time demarcated by the resignations of medical and social welfare faculty, both departments continued to assign students to the project. Highly committed and protective, the community health nurse and I tried to hold both the intent and the structure of the project constant while facilitating the work and learning of students from all three disciplines. Although we had lost the context and role model of an interdisciplinary faculty, we valued the continued interdisciplinary engagement of the students and the services they provided residents. After a year of holding sole responsibility for all three disciplines, however, the dean of the school of nursing called for a halt. The interdisciplinary project as originally conceived was ended.

UNDERSTANDING THE DEMISE OF THE PROJECT

It took outside intervention to terminate the project. It's taken four years to attain clarity and understanding of the forces and process that led to the demise of such a successful venture. Hindsight and emotional distance allow recognition of the futility of our last-ditch efforts and the significance of our not recognizing and accepting that the project had moved far off center from its original intent. The tenacity with which we hung on in the face of overwhelming responsibility and insufficient support demonstrates that we too had adopted more traditional patterns of role behavior—as women and as nurses. It also demonstrates the incredible difficulty of termination. Though we taught and encouraged our students, we had forgotten to learn the lesson of termination ourselves.

What led to the project's demise? This paper reveals many clues by describing our process and the dilemmas we faced. Over and over again, the adage "hind-sight is 20–20" has served to describe my own process of understanding. At the time, however, my focus and attention centered on creating a rich and varied clinical experience. I had not the distance, educator's maturity, nor an understanding of the historical inception of the project sufficient to attune to the forces that were leading to the project's demise.

The resignation of a covert leader certainly proved critical in precipitating the project's demise. Why could it not survive such a loss? Prior process and the loss of other individuals surely played a part. Perhaps more significant, however, was the lack of a structure or entity that transcended the individuals involved. Survival of any system requires a structure that fosters and supports continuation. Survival also requires ongoing and external nurturing and commitment.

Although the project evolved from the visions of agency leaders and administrators, no one agency owned or claimed it. The administrators rather turned their vision of the project over to a faculty recruited for their expertise and excitement at the venture. The group members, especially given the context of crisis, solidified quickly and then set about creating and nurturing the project according to their own vision, shaping it through the experiences of students and residents.

From the beginning, the project proved a collaborative venture—in its creation, its evolution, and in its day-to-day operation. Although exciting and ground-breaking, this approach resulted in no group or individual serving as overseer or one attending to the evolution and direction of the project in order to assure its continuity and clarity of purpose. No group or individual evaluated the process and outcome of the project by looking back to its mission and purpose nor forward to its future and evolution. Not having an overseer created an atmosphere of freedom which fostered creativity and flexibility in responding to forces and needs, but the benefits remained only as long as the team remained intact.

The norm and covert expectation, established early in the project's life, of "finding your own replacement" precluded any reinvolvement of administration in more than a perfunctory way. As new administrators arrived, they were apprised of the project. All supported it in concept though none became directly involved nor did they question or attend to our history, purpose, or direction. They rather condoned our continued work and involvement while making no ongoing, overt commitment of staff or resources. Neither did we expect or demand commitment or involvement. We were our own insulated, isolated, well-functioning entity.

Our experience leads to a key question that should face anyone involved in activism and creating alternative or new modes of being. When and how do you institutionalize a concept or dream? The project's demise teaches an important lesson for those who desire to go beyond the adrenaline surge and excitement of initial creation, or for those who give birth to an entity that warrants continuation. Birth is not enough. For a vision or dream to survive and thrive requires commitment and structure that transcends individuals.

Activism, that force from which the project was born, involves a process of taking positive, direct, and, most often, innovative action. Activism requires vision, creativity, tenacious dedication, and a willingness to take risks in the face of a multitude of inhibiting forces. The strong will and vision of an individual or small group provides its initial energy and direction. Institutionalize too early and you stifle potential for true innovation. Institutionalize too late, and the fruits of spontaneity and creativity may have already withered or changed in response to outside pressures calling for a return to traditionalism and stability. Fail to institutionalize and the creation either dies or wanders unconnected and undirected.

Perhaps the pearls of wisdom gleaned from this entire experience lie in the simplicity of the following advice on community building and activism:

Take the risk to fulfill a vision—to create something new.

Walk into it with your eyes open knowing there will be many forces tempting and driving you back toward a more traditional path.

Keep your eyes open—looking both back from whence you have come, forward to where you are going, and sideways to attend to what is around you.

If you have created something dear, hold it close and create an environment that will nurture its growth and continued development.

Be watchful of changes. Attend to their meaning and direction.

When it is time, dare to let go.

For in endings, there may be new beginnings.

REFERENCES

Fournier, M., & Stedman, R. (1982, September). *Learning community organization and clinical services: An interdisciplinary practicum with the elderly.* Paper presented at the meeting of the 4th National Conference on Interdisciplinary Health Care Teams, Lexington, KY.

Hawken, P. (1990, December). *Letter.* In NLN program, *"Curriculum revolution: Community building and activism."* New York: National League for Nursing.

8

Nursing in South Africa:
Black Women Organize

Nonceba Lubanga

The theme of the National League for Nursing's Seventh National Conference on Nursing Education, "Curriculum Revolution: Community Building and Activism," is a timely topic in this chaotic and changing world. The crumbling of Eastern European regimes, the unification of Germany, the changes in the Soviet Union, and the release of Mandela after 27.5 years of imprisonment in apartheid South Africa are just a few examples. Society is not static. Nursing education should be relevant to society, serve a purpose, and promote its own interests. Even in South Africa, where confusion and violence often prevail, where there are many different voices within the liberation struggle, nursing is part of this activism. The many voices create debate, and it is through this debate that South African people will be able to clarify their ideas.

To set the tone for this chapter on the black nurses' struggle in

---

This chapter is a shortened version of a work to be published in *Women and Health in Africa,* edited by Meredith Turshen and published by Africa World Press, Inc., Trenton, NJ.

South Africa, I quote Jean Watson, who, during last year's sixth national conference said, "We cannot simply change nursing, or nursing education, we must change society, our morality and our values. We must transform our worldview" (Watson, 1989).

How I wish this were the South African nursing philosophy. The South African nursing organizations, whose officials are predominately white, see themselves as an exclusive group whose interests are identical with those of the ruling class and the government in power. Africans have no influence on those who make the laws since they do not have the right to vote. Nowhere is this lack of power and influence more evident than in the case of black nurses. My intention in this chapter is to present the black nurses' perspective of how the apartheid laws of discrimination have affected their profession. Nurses occupy a key position in health care delivery and without them, the mass of health services would not be possible. Nurses are the largest group of health care providers in South Africa, as is shown in Tables 8–1, 8–2, and 8–3:

It is often argued that despite the strength and power that the nursing sector potentially wields, nurses remain largely apathetic, because they see themselves as being part of an elite profession

Table 8-1
Number of Nurses Registered as Practicing
in the South African Nursing Association
(March 1989-March 1990)

CATEGORY	1989	1990
Assistant Nurses	41,469	43,643
Enrolled Nurses	19,108	20,881
Registered Nurses	62,017	64,229
Subtotal	122,594	128,753
Nurses in Training	19,174	18,080
TOTAL	141,768	146,833

Source: Hospital and Nursing Yearbook for Southern Africa, 1990,
p. 79. Capetown: Engelhardt & Co.

Table 8-2
Number of Medical Personnel
in South Africa (1986)

Doctors	20,229
Dentists	3,486

Source: South African Institute of Race
Relations Survey, 1988/1989,
p. 3. Johannesburg: Author.

isolated from community struggles. Thus, they have been unable to bring about change in South Africa, in either the health sector or society at large, despite their numerical advantage. Some of the explanation for the nurses' apathy, the argument goes, lies in the militaristic origins of nursing as exemplified by the career of Florence Nightingale.

Nursing leaders in South Africa have actively discouraged nurses from becoming politically involved and challenging the apartheid health care system. They have repeatedly invoked notions of professional neutrality to justify this attitude. According to these leaders, the nurse's professional image must be maintained at all costs despite any social, economic, or political changes (Jacox, 1971).

That nurses, particularly black nurses in South Africa, can remain neutral while their children are shot and killed in the streets by the South African Defense Force and police and while their husbands, friends, and relatives are in jail or exile, is ludicrous to say the least.

Table 8-3
Doctor/Population Ratios (1982)

Rural	1:25,000
Urban	1:750

Source: Annual Report of the Department of
Health and Welfare, December 31,
1982

HISTORICAL OVERVIEW
OF THE BLACK NURSES' STRUGGLE

African women worked initially as domestics in South Africa's growing cities because they encountered the least resistance from men and women of other racial groups in this kind of work, and because, in the context of South Africa's racist society in which every white family aspires to have a servant, there was an ever-growing demand. In Johannesburg and other centers, the churches set up Native Girls Industrial Schools, in which girls were taught the rudiments of housekeeping. By the 1920s female African domestic servants were becoming the norm in the Rand and other urban centers.

African women with this rudimentary training could also work as domestics in hospitals and clinics. In both urban and rural areas, hospitals and clinics for Africans were largely established on the initiative of missionaries and were run by African women under the supervision of mission doctors and nurses. In 1908, Cecilia Makiwane was the first African woman to qualify as a professional nurse; she trained at Victoria Hospital in the Eastern Cape. It took another 20 years before three African women qualified as nurses and midwives at McCord's Hospital in Natal. Few African women had the educational qualifications to apply for nursing certification, and many public authorities were reluctant to provide training for them because they believed that black women were not capable of passing the nursing examination ("Origins of Contemporary Nursing," 1988).

As late as 1948 there were only some 800 African trained nurses. Unlike the situation among Afrikaners, the status of black nurses in their own communities was extremely high, despite low pay, and they had an influence in the African community out of proportion to their numbers ("Origins," 1988).

The first training courses for nurses were run by Sister Henrietta Stockdale at Kimberley Hospital in 1877. In 1913, the South African Trained Nurses' Association (SATNA) was formed. The association's original aims were to promote the professional interests of nurses and to suppress the practice of nursing by unqualified persons ("Ten Years," 1989/1990). SATNA also provided a forum for holding social gatherings, discussing pension schemes, and seeking international recognition along with similar organizations (Searle, 1965). These are nobel aims for the nursing profession, but strange to say, the African trained nurse could not be part of this association. One can see in this policy the shortsightedness of segregation and the tragedy of South Africa's racist policies. Kuper (1965, p. 217) observes that "Nursing bestows on an African woman new opportunities for freedom of individual development, but carries the burden of added responsibilities. It brings them past the threshold of Western knowledge, but shuts the door of equality in their faces."

Bantu Nurses Association

Realizing they could not belong to the SATNA, the African nurses, led by a graduate nurse from Victoria Hospital at Lovedale, decided as early as the 1920s to form their own organization, the Bantu Nurses Association (BNA). In 1930, hospitals in and around Johannesburg were training African nurses, and the white matrons (directors of nursing) held a meeting to discuss the feasibility of forming an association like the BNA. Cowles (1933, p. 233) recalls how they decided it would be better to "lay emphasis upon the formation of Wayfarer detachments (i.e., Girl Scouts) than institute an association." The matrons thought that the Witwatersrand Branch of SATNA should elect one of its (white) members to represent Bantu nurses. SATNA officials thwarted and stalled the African nurses' efforts to form their own organization until November 1932, when they finally allowed the BNA to be affiliated with the SATNA.

The BNA was more active than Borcherds (1958) would have us believe. Black nurses all over South Africa, including one working in Southwest Africa (now Namibia), manifested great interest in the BNA (Cowles, 1933). The chief aims of the BNA were not much different from those of the SATNA except that the BNA also hoped to gain the confidence of the African people and be of service to them. The BNA grew, and by 1941 it had seven branches, a national headquarters, officers, and was holding national conferences (Wright, 1985).

South African Nursing Association

In the early 1940s, South Africa faced a severe nursing crisis. Contributing factors were poor living conditions, low salaries, a shortage of nurses, restrictions on married nurses, and nurses leaving the profession ("Origins," 1988). The withdrawal of 1,100 registered nurses from civilian services to staff military hospitals both locally and abroad during World War II exacerbated the shortage of nurses. As no African nurses were trained to occupy high ranking posts, none were sent abroad at this time (Searle, 1965). SATNA could not help nurses meet the crisis because of its undemocratic structure, aims, and objectives.

As a direct result of dissatisfaction with SATNA, white nurses started a movement in 1942 to form a new organization along trade union lines (Borcherds, 1958) Searle(1965) notes:

> This organization convened a meeting in the Red Cross Hall, Johannesburg, on 30th August, 1942, with a view to organizing the Nursing profession as a Trade Union . . . the main speaker was a representative of the Garment Worker's Union. He stressed the fact that nurses were exploited by their employers (a statement which was unfortunately too true) and many of the long suffering nurses immediately reacted favourably to this sympathetic technique. [p. 248]

One or two radical medical practitioners spoke about the exploitation of student nurses, who were the main source of labor, but who received neither adequate salaries nor proper tuition.

In response to what became known as the "trade union crisis of 1942," the established leadership of SATNA and the Department of Public Health rapidly joined forces. The matron-in-chief of the South African Military Nursing Service, released the organizing secretary of SATNA to undertake a tour of all branches of the association and address mass meetings of nurses on the subject of trade unions. During these meetings, speakers warned nurses that the political aura associated with unions was contrary to the spirit of nursing (Searle, 1965).

What worried both the government and the SATNA leadership was the thought that nurses might adopt a trade union mentality and might even be persuaded to strike to improve their situation. Because of the possibility that Afrikaner nurses would branch off from SATNA and form their own separate association and rumors that Afrikaner nationalists intended to make the reform of nursing a plank in their 1943 election platform, the government gave the 1943 Nursing Bill priority (Marks, 1988; "Origins," 1988). Trade unionists believed that if they had the nurses on their side, they would have the government where they wanted it, because "no government could withstand the political pressure which the withholding of nursing services would exert on them" (Searle, 1965, p. 251).

SATNA campaigned vigorously for a closed shop professional association and their own governing body. All of their previous efforts had failed, but on this occasion they were successful. The South African Nursing Act No. 45 of 1944, initially introduced to the House of Assembly as a private measure by Margaret Ballinger, was taken over by the government and passed as a government measure (Borcherds, 1958). The South African Nursing Association (SANA) replaced SATNA as the professional association to which all registered nurses, student nurses, and midwives, regardless of color, were now compelled to belong. (Under section 38 of the [1978] Nursing Amendment Act No. 50, nurses of all categories who are practicing in South Africa are still required to be members. Failure to comply constitutes improper or disgraceful conduct, which is liable to penalties ranging from a caution or reprimand to removal of the nurse's name from the register of practicing nurses [Strauss, 1981].) SANA's objectives were to raise the status, maintain the integrity, and promote the interests of the nursing profession in South Africa by becoming nursing's representative to government, provincial, and local authorities in regard to employment conditions, salaries, leave, and pensions (Searle, 1965). With the creation of SANA, the BNA was effectively eliminated.

According to "Origins" (1988, p. 8) "the non-racialism of the 1944 Nursing Act seemed to represent a more liberal mood" than that prevailing at the creation of the segregated SATNA in 1913. Unity between nurses of different class, racial, and ethnic origins was a real, if superficial, possibility in 1944, given the liberal climate of the war years and the small numbers of black trained nurses. Even at that time, there were those who contested the achievements of the 1944 Act. "Origins" (1988) noted that Charlotte Searle, then Director of Nursing in the Transvaal and already a dominant figure in the SANA and South African Nursing Council (SANC), was explicit on the reasons. She argued that "non-European nurses" were only included on an equal basis in the 1944 Act because at that time there were very few of them and because the nurses were assured by the provincial authorities responsible for hospital services, that the authorities did not intend training black nurses for full certification:

> If we had known at the time that the policy of the provincial authorities was just the opposite we, and I for one, would certainly not have agreed to the introduction of the Bill as it was introduced in 1944. We would have fought it to the last ditch. We certainly would not have liked to do something which would ultimately have wrecked the European nursing services in South Africa. At any event, because there was no problem at the time, it was decided that there would be no color bar. [Report of the Select Committee on Nursing, 1954, paragraph 313, p. 153]

SANA developed a highly bureaucratic structure that stifled progress within the organization. Nurses continued to express their discontent in the form of strikes, despite the SANA constraints. Black nurses working at the Alexandra Clinic in Alexandra Township just outside Johannesburg went on strike in 1947. The clinic's board of managers claimed not to know what the grievances were. Cowles commented from the United States, on the basis of news from her friends, that the whole affair had resulted from intimidation by the "communists" who had stirred up the community (Wright, 1985). What is surprising about Cowles' reaction to the nurses' strike is that she herself marveled that nurses did not complain about the horrible working conditions, long working hours, and poor salaries. The Alexandra strike was a prelude to others that followed.

Nursing Strikes Continue

In 1949, the student nurses at Victoria Hospital in Lovedale (a part of Alice, Cape Province) went on strike to protest the unfair dismissal of a nurse who had presented a petition of grievances to the hospital administration. One complaint concerned the composition of the hospital board: hospital authorities had appointed two board members to represent the nurses. The nurses felt that they did not have a voice, that the appointed individuals represented not their interests but the interests of the hospital authorities who had selected them. Phyllis P. Jordan recalls the strike:

> Going on strike was a tough moral issue, for it involved withholding needed services to their patients. After a long debate on this question, the [student] nurses decided to boycott the hospital and its facilities, but report for duty in the wards as scheduled. Even though a number of staff nurses were with the trainees in spirit, it was decided that they would not strike. Then the nurses walked out of the dormitories, the dining halls, and the classrooms. They camped on an open field just outside the hospital and went to the wards only on duty. This meant no beds, no blankets, no food, and no laundry services for them.

> When the communities around the hospital heard that the nurses were out on strike, they rallied around the strikers. Students at Fort Hare University, senior students at Lovedale, and some Lovedale teachers such as Mr. Mac Sipho Makhalima and the late Victor Hermanus brought mattresses, blankets, and groceries. Some wives of the African staff members at Fort Hare pitched in too with pots, pans, and food. The women from Ntselamanzi, Gqumashe, Dyhamala, and Gaga—the villages around these campuses—came in to help with the cooking and the laundry.

> Coordinating all these efforts were Mrs. Mzamane, wife of Professor Mzamane at Fort Hare, and Mrs. Xhaphile, wife of the Principal's secretary at Fort Hare. These women literally left their houses and children to attend to the needs of the striking nurses. From Lovedale came Tazana Mali and her sister Nonke

Mali, a cook at Elukhanyisweni, Fort Hare. The laundry service organized by Mrs. Mzamane and Mrs. Xhaphile ran as smoothly as though there were no strike, and this was in the days when none of them had washing machines. Their resolve was that these nurses had to be clean every time they went on duty, and they had to be fed.

The women did a marvelous job. Mac Sipho Makhalima kept up the nurses' spirits on cold nights, playing his piano accordion. Sometimes the people sang and he accompanied them, and sometimes they just listened to Mac playing.

After two weeks of drawn out struggle, the issue was resolved and the nurses went back to work. [personal communication, August 1989]

The story of the Victoria Hospital strike shows how women can display great courage when roused to action, courage that is often greater than that of men because women frequently have immediate responsibility for children at home. It also demonstrates the solidarity that existed between nurses and the community and contradicts the notion that nurses are an elite group, totally isolated from their communities. Would the local people at Alice, and the students and teachers at Fort Hare and Lovedale have rallied around isolated elites?

Separate Registers

The coming to power of the National Party in 1948 had a number of effects on nursing. Black nurses had always been discriminated against, for despite equal training their salaries were far lower than those of whites, and their training facilities were inferior. To foster apartheid in the nursing profession, the Nursing Act of 1957 was passed. Prior to 1957, legislation relating to trained nurses and midwives was not instituted along racial lines. Under the 1957 Act, separate registers were created for the different ethnic groups, namely Africans, colored/Asians, and whites. Black nurses were barred from holding office on the central board of the SANA (Sutton, 1986).

Marsha Resha, an African nurse who was in the opposition leadership, described the situation in this way:

> In 1956, on hearing about the pending bill which would amend the 1944 Nursing Act, to create separate registers along racial lines, African and European nurses around the Transvaal area had several meetings to discuss its merits. There were heated arguments between black and white nurses. The white nurses tried to convince the black nurses that apartheid was good for them and that since it was the country's new policy there was nothing wrong with creating separate registers in SANC and SANA. Realizing the futility of their pleas and of trying to reason with the white nurses, the African nurses decided to form the Rand Nurses Professional Club, which was later instrumental in creating the Federation of South African Nurses and Midwives (FOSANAM). [personal communication, July 1989]

According to Marks (1988, p. 36), "The passage of the 1957 Nursing Act roused passionate opposition among black and a handful of white nurses. To add insult to injury, the state attempted to use the new registration forms to force the much hated pass system on African nurses in order to use them as an example for other African women who were resisting the extension of the pass laws at the time." (The pass system required blacks to carry at all times a "passbook" containing the person's identity and employment record. Failure to produce the "passbook" when requested by a police officer was a criminal offense.)

This policy was much resented by nonwhite nurses, particularly African women, because in order to obtain their identity numbers they had to report to officials of the Native Affairs Department, who were liable to issue "passbook/reference" books to them. They also objected to stating their race as "Native."

Resha recalls the nurses' response to the threat of being used by the government for the extension of pass laws:

> Between 1955 and 1956, many nurses joined the Women's League of the African National Congress (ANC) and the

Federation of South African Women. The Nursing Council was instructed by the government to write to the matrons of the hospital requiring all the nurses to produce I.D. numbers. So, the Rand Nurses Professional Club elected me to go to the Native Affairs Department offices in Pretoria to inquire about the I.D. numbers. After being driven from pillar to post in these offices, I finally landed a clerk who told me that the only way I would have an I.D. number would be for me to get a "passbook."

The matrons, knowing the amount of resistance to carrying "passbooks" by women, never had the courage to tell the nurses that by asking them to produce I.D. numbers for registration they meant "passbooks." Realizing that the hospital officials tried to trick them into getting the "passes," the nurses were seething with anger. They took the matter to the Federation of South African Women and Women's League of the ANC and briefed them on the problems of the pass system and how it would interfere with their day-to-day work with their patients. Some of the problems they pointed out were: constant harassment by police and being searched for "passes.," which would result in lateness for work; absenteeism resulting from being arrested if one forgot to carry the "pass" on one's person; and disruption of their daily lives at home by constant police night raids making them psychologically and emotionally unfit to work effectively with their patients the following day.

The Federation of South African Women, the Women's League of the ANC, and the nurses organized a big demonstration of over 500 women and marched to Baragwanath Hospital, where they met with the matrons and explained their reasons for resisting the proposed legislation. The matrons wrote back to the Nursing Council and the proposal was withdrawn for the time being. The next group of women to be victimized were the domestic workers, whose employers simply loaded them in their cars and then took them to "pass" offices where they were issued "passes." [personal communication, July 1989]

Protest meetings took place at many hospitals. At a meeting of nonwhite nurses held in January 1955 at King Edward VIII Hospital in Durban, tempers rose to such an extent that the police were summoned, but the women had quieted down by the time the police arrived. The hospital superintendent then announced that the Nursing Council had informed him that African women nurses who were not in possession of their identity numbers need not furnish them (*South African Institute of Race Relations Survey,* 1958–1959).

Nonwhite nurses at Johannesburg's Baragwanath Hospital also held protest meetings and announced that they would refuse to complete the forms. According to the (Johannesburg) *Star* (March 22, 1958), the Federation of South African Women decided to arrange a demonstration in support of the nurses. The authorities feared that disturbances might result. The African townships were cordoned off from the hospital, roadblocks were set up, the police assembled in strength in the roads leading to the hospital, and it was reported that a ward had been cleared for possible casualties. As a result of the precautions taken, the police probably outnumbered the demonstrators who arrived at the hospital.

Resha described the formation of the protest organization, the Federation of South African Nurses and Midwives:

> In 1957, when the Nursing Bill was being debated in Parliament, nursing administrators and matrons were summoned to Cape Town to testify to the Select Committee that Africans were inferior and unsuitable to have the same nursing profession as whites. The African nurses, who were still members of the same association with voting rights, sent memoranda to the Select Committee expressing their opposition to the proposed legislation. They were ignored.

> This led to the formation of the Federation of South African Nurses and Midwifes (FOSANAM), which was launched in Johannesburg in 1957, even before the bill creating separate registers for nurses became an act. It was a protest organization of predominantly black nurses and a few whites, with strong branches on the Reef, Cape Town, Alice, Transkei, and other parts of the Eastern Cape Province. Nurses from Natal and the Orange Free State joined the federation at a later stage. With their slogan "disease knows no color," the nurses protested the introduction of segregation into their profession. They knew what had happened when the Bantu

Education Act was introduced in 1954 and that the same was going to happen to their noble profession.

The government had anticipated opposition and, as in the case of Bantu education, had dangled sops all over and by stringent legislation made it well-nigh impossible for any nurse practicing and/or in training to follow her profession unless she was registered in the proper ethnic registers and in the case of Africans had a "pass" for I.D.

For the first time in the annals of the nursing profession in South Africa, African nurses were promoted to senior staff positions in almost all the clinics and hospitals that served an African clientele. A number of those promoted were the charter members of FOSANAM. The women had long deserved these promotions, for they were excellent health providers, their reputations beyond dispute. Co-opted now into the new structures, they were compromised and could not carry on their protests. [personal communication, July 1989]

Contrary to what is written about how FOSANAM died in its infancy, Resha maintains that, in fact, it had branches all over South Africa and had international support as well. The federation held its third conference in Orlando, Transvaal in 1961. Unfortunately, as Resha noted earlier, the media completely ignored coverage of these events.

An editorial comment in the *Lancet* ("Apartheid in Nursing," 1957) highlighted the dangers and the implications of the 1957 Nursing Act. It also pointed out that, apart from its own leading article on the subject, there was virtually no coverage in the press. A circular to key members of the Royal College of Nursing and the National Council of Nurses mentioned the new act briefly. Whyte (1957), writing in a British journal called *Nursing Times,* was the only reader to demand more information.

1960s to the 1990s

The nurses' struggle for improved working conditions and their protests against unjust policies within various health institutions continued unabated despite lack of support from official nursing organizations such as SANA. The alternative to SANA, in which membership is compulsory, would logically be a trade union. South African nurses were able to join unions that represented them as employees in certain situations; however, they were strongly discouraged from doing so ("Warning," 1983).

The kind of intimidation to which union-minded nurses were subjected was demonstrated in the 1961 nurses' strike at King George Tuberculosis Hospital in Durban. According to Luckhardt and Wall (1980), the strike was called to protest an incident in which the matron of the nurses' residence severely caned 12 student nurses, allegedly for arriving in class a few minutes late. Skilled and unskilled hospital workers supported the nurses' demand for the expulsion of the matron.

With assistance from the local Hospital Workers' Union, the nurses made several other demands. They wanted the policy of unequal eating facilities abolished. The African nurses were given lower quality meals, were required to bring their own eating utensils, and paid more than whites for their board and lodging. They demanded raises in their scandalously low salaries. They demanded extension of maternity leave to unmarried pregnant women in order to prevent fatal illegal abortions. They wanted an unemployment insurance fund. They demanded an end to the degrading practice that required African employees to make a cross when collecting their paychecks, instead of signing for them. Finally, they wanted African nurses to receive the same prophylactic treatment against tuberculosis that was given to all other employees (Luckhardt & Wall, 1980).

The nurses received support from local and international communities. Some of their demands were met, but the hospital superintendent refused to fire the matron. Twenty-two of the striking nurses were fired, and all nurses were threatened with dismissal if they belonged to a union. Nursing authorities argued that trade unions could not act on behalf of nurses with regard to conditions of service or what professional acts the nurses might perform because these were the functions of SANA. Yet it took a trade union to help nurses at King George Tuberculosis Hospital improve their working conditions.

In some countries, nurses engage in collective bargaining and are organized either in associations or trade unions to bargain collectively for better conditions of employment and nursing standards. The American Nurses' Association established an economic security program in 1946 that was designed to enable state and local associations to bargain for their members (Stern, 1982). In England, the Royal College of Nursing is the professional association that won certification as an independent trade union in 1977, and it is the collective bargaining body for nurses there. British nurses are also represented by trade unions that are affiliated with the Trade Union Congress (Salvage, 1985). In Australia, the Royal Australian Nursing Federation is affiliated with the Australian council of trade unions and is the collective bargaining body for nurses there (Gardner & McCoppin, 1986). In South Africa, the 1978 Nursing Amendment Act (No. 50) made strike action by nurses a statutory offense with fines of up to 500 South African rand, one year in jail, or both ("Warning," 1983).

The 1978 Act provided for a nonracial nursing council to represent South African citizens; this provision effectively excluded many registered African nurses who, in terms of South African law, were citizens of independent homelands. African nurses actively opposed forced segregation into separate white nurses' domination of *SANA* ("Historical Overview," 1988).

When these homeland nursing associations were formed, the African nurses who worked in the homelands or the so-called independent states received no financial assistance from SANA even though they had been paying annual dues to this body for decades. They had to start afresh to build their associations. Most nurses in the homelands subscribe to a homeland association as well as SANA so as to keep SANA membership in case they need to work in South Africa at some point.

Despite the 1978 legislation, the 1980s brought many changes. Following the waves of trade union activism that began in 1973, hospital workers organized in Natal, the Transvaal, and the Cape. They joined such unions as the Black Health and Allied Workers Union, the General and Allied Workers Union, the National Education Health and Allied Workers Union, and the Baragwanath Health Workers Association. The unions aimed to break down barriers between different grades of health workers by bringing all hospital workers together in one organization, regardless of their skills and levels of training. These unions represented health workers in a wave of hospital strikes that began in the Transvaal with the action at Baragwanath, the showcase hospital in Soweto that serves a population of two million blacks.

In August 1985, *City Press* (Johannesburg) reported that 16 nurses, picked from Baragwanath's "cream of the crop," were transferred to the Johannesburg General Hospital to take care of white patients. Hospital administrators took this move to ease the nursing shortage that threatened the white hospital's services. An investigation carried out by the Baragwanath Health Workers Association discovered that the nurses were not consulted prior to their transfer and that most of them were forced to go to Johannesburg. The (Johannesburg) *Star* alleged that skilled and experienced African nurses were being drawn from Baragwanath, which has a bed occupancy rate of over 100 percent (cited in "Historical Overview," 1988). The highly trained nurses were angry because they felt that their skills were equally important for black patients who were already at a disadvantage. The Baragwanath Health Workers Association said it was "totally immoral and unacceptable" to use selected health personnel to upgrade the services of certain communities (*City Press,* August 8, 1988).

Although nurses are allowed to join unions, the Nursing Act of 1978 forbids them to go on strike or take part in demonstrations or sit-ins. In South Africa, health workers have no established collective bargaining rights. As working conditions continue to deteriorate with government funding cutbacks, nurses continue to defy SANA and confront health officials. One of the issues that is presently being challenged by the nurses is the requirement by certain hospital authorities (e.g., Baragwanath Hospital) that they either lose weight or lose their jobs. It was apparently alleged that overweight nurses "fall asleep on the job" ("Ten Years," 1989/1990, p. 50). Nurses, together with other health workers, are demanding desegregation of health services to ease the overburdened black public hospitals and to end racist employment practices. These include temporary employees since such workers have little job security and are grossly discriminated against compared to permanent workers (mainly the more highly educated white workers) who enjoy a degree of security and receive significant benefits. Temporary workers are subject to only 24 hours notice of dismissal even if they have worked for a lifetime (*South African Labour Bulletin,* 1990).

In terms of the Nursing Amendment Act, strike action by nurses is a statutory offense subject to penalties of up to 500 South African rands, one year in jail, or both. Several nurses across the country who participated in strikes from 1987 to 1990 have been charged. This has brought into focus the apartheid mentality which prevails in South Africa's health care establishment, despite apparent liberalization.

SANC, the statutory body which rules on individual nurses' credentials, has summoned the nurses who face these charges for disciplinary action for "improper and disgraceful conduct." If found guilty, their registration may be withdrawn.

As the largest group of skilled health workers, South African nurses, black and white, have a crucial role in transforming the present health care system. First, they must develop progressive nursing associations that will help create a primary health care approach which emphasizes the importance of self-reliance and community activism and decision making.

REFERENCES

Apartheid in Nursing. (1957, June 8). *Lancet,* 1182.

Borcherds, M. G. (1958, July). The South African Nursing Act: An account of events leading up to and subsequent to the passing of the South African Nursing Act No. 69 of 1957. *International Nursing Review,* 33.

Cowles, R. (1933). The Bantu Nurses' Association. *South African Nursing Record, 20,* 233.

Gardner, H., & McCoppin, B. (1986). Vocation, career, or both? Politicalization of Australian Nurses, Victoria 1984–1986. *Australian Journal of Advanced Nursing, 4,* 24–35.

Historical overview of nursing organization in South Africa. (1988, October). *Critical Health, 55–59*.

Hospital and nursing yearbook for southern Africa (30th revised ed.). (1990). Capetown: H. Engelhardt & Co.

Jacox, A. (1971). Collective action and control of practice by professionals. *Nursing Forum, 10,* 239–257.

Kuper, L. (1965). *An African bourgeoise: Race, class and politics in South Africa.* New Haven and London: Yale University Press.

Luckhardt, K., & Wall, B. (1980). *Organize or starve! The history of the South African Congress of Trade Unions.* New York: International Publishers.

Marks, S. (1988, May). *Class, race, and gender in the South African nursing profession.* Paper presented to the Canadian Association of African Studies, Queen's University, Kingston, Ontario.

The Nursing Bill: What it means to nurses. (1978). *Nursing News, 1,* 1.

Origins of contemporary nursing organization in South Africa. (1988, October). *Critical Health,* 5–9.

Salvage, J. (1985). *The politics of nursing.* London: Heineman.

Searle, C. (1965). *The history of the development of nursing in South Africa 1952–1960.* Cape Town: Struik.

South African Institute of Race Relations Survey. (1958/1959). *South Afican Labour Bulletin, 15*(1), 173.

South African Institute of Race Relations Survey. (1988/1989). *Number of medical personnel in South Africa, 1986.* Johannesburg: Author.

South African Labour Bulletin. (1990). *15*(1).

Stern, E. (1982). Collective Bargaining: Means of conflict resolution. *Nursing Administration Quarterly, 6, 2.*

Strauss, S. A. (1981). Legal handbook and health personnel. Cape Town: King Edward VII Trust, 24–37.

Sutton, R. V. (1986). Professional Association Versus Trade Unions. *Nursing Republic of South Africa, 1,* 14–15.

Ten years in the health struggle. (1989/1990). *Critical Health* (special edition), *29,* 4.

Warning against pitfalls of a trade union. (1983). *Nursing News, 7,* 1.

Watson, J. (1989). Paper presented at the National League for Nursing Sixth National Conference on Nursing Education, Philadelphia, December 6–9, 1989.

Wright, M. (1985). *Health activism in Southern Africa: Nurses and primary health care.* Proceedings of the First Workshop of the Project, Poverty, Health and the State in Southern Africa, p. 7. Columbia University, New York, November 1985.

Whyte, B. (1957, July 12). *Nursing Times,* 786.

9

Creating Communities of Caring

Sister M. Simone Roach

A number of words and phrases in the conference program have been used to communicate a powerful message. These words and phrases include community building; reclaiming our communities; mobilizing the nursing community's strength, expertise, compassion and vision; exploring new possibilities. We have spoken of revolution and transformation, emancipatory power. All of this has been presented, as Patty Hawken says in the conference program, in the context of the "extraordinary opportunity to address the many pressing ills of our current system: the AIDS epidemic, the homeless, the need for more primary care and care for the chronically ill elderly" (1990, p. B).

The actual design of the conference has provided for broad input and professional sharing, for story and narrative. Much has transpired, but many interchanges will go unrecorded, particularly the personal conversations we have had with each other over the past few days. It is my hope that all of this will change our lives—how we think, respond, and design our plans for the future. This conference, and the context in which it has been planned and executed, is a vivid mirroring of our heritage, of who we have been

123

traditionally, and who we are called to be now as a profession dedicated to the service of others.

In our nursing literature, we talk about the slavery of a limited vision, objectification of students to ends predetermined by behavioral goals. We propose, as antidote, teacher-student partnerships, flexibility, and commitment to individual differences. We appeal to the need for a new worldview of educational practices, for social responsibility—an interpretative stance, with the intent to unveil, understand, and critique beliefs and assumptions. These assumptions, we assert, include the assumptions implicit in the rational, technological epistemology of practice; medicocentrism, a narrow biomedical view focusing on disease rather than illness; gender bias; cultural supremacy of theoretical knowledge; relationships of dominance, the oppression of a model of teaching which relates to students as receptacles (the banking concept). From, and in all of this, we see the need for emancipation.

There is one theme, hidden if not deliberately excluded in our literature. This theme has to do with the violence we do to ourselves in overwork, in stretching ourselves to the limit as teachers, researchers, spouses, parents, and in all the other roles we assume in our generous day-to-day giving. What is so regrettable about this is our failure to understand the meaning of reciprocity and its manifestation in our resistance to being cared for by others.

THE CULTURAL CONTEXT

As I reflect on the curriculum revolution to which we are committed, I am reminded that this phenomenon needs to be situated within the context of a larger cultural ethos. This is the culture of Western society of which we are the beneficiaries, and alas, the victims as well. There are elements within this culture that are in competition with, and are antithetical to, what we are trying to call forth in nursing today. In order to realize the scope and revolutionary character of our commitment, we need a clearer view of the challenge and the resistance emanating from prevailing cultural values.

One concrete illustration of the impact of the cultural ethos is reflected in a recent 20-year study of the values and career preferences of freshmen entering colleges in this country. (Cooperative Institutional Research Program, 1985).

> Most of the value items on the annual freshmen survey showing increases in recent years are concerned with money, power, and status: being well-off financially, being an authority, having administrative responsibility for others, and obtaining recognition. . . . In contrast, values showing the largest declines involve altruistic activities and social concerns: helping others, promoting racial understanding, cleaning up the environment, participating in community action programs, and keeping up with political affairs. . . . Increased student interest in career-specific majors such as business has been accompanied by rising materialistic and power values, while decreased student interest in education, social science, the arts, humanities, nursing, social work, allied health, and the clergy is reflected in declining altruism and social concern. [p. 2]

Predominant values of our cultural ethos are also revealed in critiques by 20th century prophets who have been nudging our consciences over the past several decades. Not the least of these, Pitirim Sorokin, one-time Dean of Sociology at Harvard University, portrays our culture as a culture in crisis. In one of his many volumes, *Crisis of Our Age* (1942), Sorokin characterizes this crisis as one of extraordinary proportions.

> It is not merely an economic or political maladjustment, but involves simultaneously almost the whole of Western culture and society, in all their main sectors. It is a crisis in their art and science, philosophy and religion, law and morals, manners and mores; in the forms of social, political, and economic organization, including the nature of the family and marriage—in brief, it is a crisis involving almost the whole way of life, thought, and conduct of Western society. More precisely, it consists in a disintegration of a fundamental form of Western culture and society dominant for the last four centuries. [pp. 16–17]

The crisis to which Sorokin refers involves the dissolution of the sensate culture which became dominant after the 15th century. It is the culture that has ushered in the marvelous achievements in science and technology that have been the source of a prosperity and technological progress the world has never before known. This sensate culture, however, has also been the context and the impetus for our 20th century capacity for global and ecological destruction. It is the concrete expression of a philosophy of naturalism which claims reality to be exclusively physical—what one can taste, see, feel, touch, hear, and manipulate—and asserts the only way of knowing is through the empirical method of the sciences. Sensate culture, according to Sorokin, is in crisis. It has failed because, like other dominant cultures preceding it, it has become reductionist. The sensate culture has materialized all human life and values.

Alexander Solzhenitsyn, in his commencement address at Harvard University (1978), speaks similarly about the decline in the West and points to its spiritual exhaustion, moral poverty, and "the calamity of an autonomous, irreligious humanistic consciousness" (p. 49).

In a more recent study of American society, Bellah, Madsen, Sullivan, Swidler, and Tipton (1985) note the erosion of those "social integuments" which Tocqueville (1969) claims are needed to deter the distructive potential of a growing individualism in our relationships, in family, civic, and political life.

These are predominant elements of the culture we have inherited, and of the world we shape and are shaped by. It is a culture enriched by great technological achievements with limitless capacity for future progress. It is also the source of the mechanization and the technologicalization of our lives and values. What we perceive to be the problem in education is but one imprint of a larger phenomenon which touches every aspect of our lives.

Perhaps we could rephrase our diagnosis of the problem in nursing education as the "crisis of our age," a crisis within the professions, education, nursing practice, management, and research. It is the crisis studied so thoroughly in the American schools in the 1950s. It is at the root of what we observe as the great "implosions" of the 1990s.

Over the past few months, we have witnessed the breakdown of political systems and the reshaping of the European continent. Crisis, defined as what is experienced "when one world has died; another is powerless to be born . . . of being condemned to the anxious space between the no-longer and the not-yet" (Rowe, 1980, p. 13), is that with which human beings all over the world are struggling. It would be unfortunate if we were to view our professional experience and need for a curriculum revolution outside of this national and global reality.

THE NURSING PROFESSION: A SIGN OF HOPE

What we have been observing over the past several months on the political, social, and economic scenes are implosions rather than explosions. Implosions, by definition, create vacuums. Nursing has much to bring to the "anxious space of the no-longer and the not-yet" (Rowe, 1980, p. 13). With its rich heritage, unique gifts, and professional resources, I believe nursing is called—as never before—to shape what will fill the vacuum.

Emancipation, empowerment, calling forth, "helping the other grow" (Mayeroff, 1971, p. 9), unveiling, are words and phrases we, as professionals, are trying to speak to the profession and the world around us. They are expressions of what we are all about, expressions of our human mode of being. While reflecting on the conference program, I was struck by what might be labeled the subliminal messages running through the themes and "subjectives." I would interpret the primary message as the importance of reclaiming our identity as a caring profession, mobilizing our human capacity to care within a community of human persons, and directing our energies to creatively shape health care to meet the needs of those who cry for help on a shrinking but suffering planet. This is a singularly challenging call.

Today, wonderful things are happening in the health care world because of nursing. This conference is evidence of that. On the international scene, there are many signs of hope in the vision and commitment of nurse educators, researchers, practitioners, and nurse managers who are shaping a futuristic nursing while, in the words of Patty Hawken, "reclaiming the community and mobilizing the nursing community's strength, expertise, compassion, and vision to create a new brand of health care" (1990, p. B).

Over the past four years, I have had the privilege of working in the Nursing Division of St. Boniface General Hospital in Winnipeg, Canada. This is truly an institution without walls. Through the leadership of Jan Dick, who, as Vice President of Nursing, has a gift for attracting and maintaining a staff of unusual caliber and commitment, the Nursing Division of this hospital is respected nationally and internationally for a remarkable degree of creativity and commitment to excellence in patient care. I am sure we can all name other institutions and agencies of similar quality.

At its heart, nursing is a personal service to persons in need. As a human community, we have responded to a call to service through our historical evolution from a natural human response to human need, to a vocation, to an organized profession. In essence, the challenge has been a perennial call of our humanity to reach out to those who suffer and who need our help. That is why in scholarly research, in the wisdom of the human community, and in our education and practice, we have claimed that nursing is intrinsically a manifestation of human care.

THE MANY FACES OF HUMAN CARE

Much is being done within the profession to capture the centrality of caring in nursing. Over the past decade, the International Human Caring Conferences, sponsored by the International Association for Human Caring, have become dynamic forums for sharing research and experience. I doubt anyone can participate in one of those conferences and not believe in the great potential nursing has for transforming the entire system of health care. The research and writing of many of our colleagues, including persons in this audience, express through story and dialogue how human care is at the heart of nursing practice, education, and research.

We need to shout from the housetops the primacy of caring in nursing; at the same time, it is important that we continue to study and share our reflections on caring's various entailments. We must break through the fuzziness with which caring is frequently under-stood. In reflections and research on caring, we need to more sharply name the questions. I have found it helpful to use the following categories for organizing the caring project.

1. The *ontological* category addresses the questions, what is the being of caring and what is caring in itself?

2. The *anthropological* category poses the question, what does it mean to be a caring person? Anthropology deals with the cultural concepts of caring, giving, being cared for.

3. The *ontical* category, referring to the study of some entities in relation to other entities, asks the question, "what is a person doing when he or she is caring?

4. The *epistemological* category relates to how caring can be defined and evidenced, how caring can be measured and quantified.

5. The *pedagogical* category is concerned with how caring is learned and taught.

In the few moments I have here today, I will discuss the ontological and the ontical categories and reflect upon where my journey through these categories has taken me over the past several years.

Toward an Ontology of Caring

For as long as I can recall my experience in nursing education, the concept of caring has been central or foundational in my understanding of the nature of nursing. This conviction has been affirmed over and over again by the contributions of many in the profession, including Madeleine Leininger, Jean Watson, Patricia Benner, and Nancy Diekelmann, in a list of researchers and writers that continues to grow.

Perhaps the most exciting moment in my own research on caring came with a special flash of insight, in one of those rare moments of experience, when it became very clear to me that caring is the human mode of being (1987). Caring names every human being and distinguishes none. We care, not because we are nurses, but because we are human beings. Every human being, because he or she is human, has a natural capacity, indeed, a natural need to care and be cared for. What distinguishes a nurse from a doctor, a social worker, an engineer, or a housekeeper is not that some of us care and others do not, but rather that we differ in how we express the caring capacity we all share.

The call to care is not simply an ethical imperative, i.e., it does not simply mean we ought to care, or that caring is a good thing to do. Rather, in an important sense, we *are* care. Our human mode of being is to care. We are human to the degree that we care. We become fulfilled as human beings to the extent our caring capacity is called forth, nurtured, and expressed.

The capacity to care, while it may be repressed or suppressed, is almost indestructible. Many examples of how caring seeks to manifest itself, even in the most inhumane of situations, document this claim (May, 1969; Burrell & Hauerwas, 1974; Speer, 1971). One example will suffice here.

May, reflecting on the meaning of care, refers to "a strange phenomenon about the Vietnam War" (1969, p. 284). This strange phenomenon has to do with the nature and message of photographs taken of that war; pictures of the wounded caring for each other, of soldiers taking care of the injured, of a marine with his arms around a wounded comrade—the wounded one crying out in pain and bewilderment. What comes back in the photo, notes May, is "on this elemental level, *care*" (p. 284). May describes the bewilderment equally communicated by the helpless child whose face is "dirty with the smoke and soot from the smoke bomb," (p. 284) and by the "black marine looking down at the child, commanding and somewhat hideous in his battle uniform" (p. 284). Reflecting on what may have been the thought of the marine as he experienced this situation, May says,

> I do not think (the marine) ponders these things consciously: I think he only sees there another human being with a common base of humanity on which they pause for a moment in the swamps of Vietnam. His look is care. [p. 285]

Caring is not simply an emotional feeling or attitudinal response. Caring is a total way of being, of relating, of acting; a quality of investment and engagement in the other—person, idea, project, or self as "other"—in which one expresses the self fully, and through which one touches most intimately and authentically what it means to be human.

Caring is not unique *to* nursing in that it distinguishes nursing from other professional or vocational groups; rather, caring is unique *in* nursing in the sense that, among all characteristics descriptive of nursing, caring is unique. It has primacy.

Consistent with this conceptualization of caring, then, nursing is no more and no less than the professionalization of the human capacity to care through the acquisition and use of the knowledge and skills required for nursing's prescribed roles in education, practice, research, and administration.

We have striking and convincing evidence over many years that students select nursing as a career because they want to help, to care for people. Even with the changes in value orientations and career choices among the general population of students, we still manage to recruit a core of students from a broad range of age and experience who come to us with this motivation. The challenge to nurse educators, practitioners, researchers, and nurse administrators is to tap, affirm, and call forth the student's natural capacity to care, and to provide the environment for learning and practice that facilitates its professionalization.

This insight has radical implications for teaching and learning, for practice, research, and management. I believe we as nurses know this and, in many ways, offer our support. There is, however, a gap between our beliefs and our everyday comportment. I suggest this is a complex issue, as multifaceted as the complexity of each one of us.

During the course of my research on caring, I had many ups and downs. I wrote beautiful things, gave many inspirational talks, and engaged in lively conversations with professionals and friends. On occasion my inner conflicts were so troubling, I wanted to scrap it all, relegate those carefully worded and fastidiously nuanced papers to the wastebasket. What was the problem? The problem had to do with the discrepancy I experienced between the ideals I was writing and speaking about and the reality of my everyday relationships with the people I lived and worked. Deeper and more fundamental still was my refusal to accept my own vulnerability, my own woundedness and need to be cared for. To the degree I could not acknowledge my own limitations, my own need for care, I was less free to be a caring person.

Caring involves caring for ourselves as well as others, and this sometimes requires that we allow others to enter our personal space to share our vulnerability and to heal our woundedness. As professionals, I do not believe we are very good at doing this but, if we are to create those caring environments required to set us all free, we must allow ourselves to be within a community of persons who need to be cared for by others.

Toward an Onticology of Caring

I will briefly address one of the other categories for research on caring that I noted earlier. This is the *ontical* category, which is concerned with entities, or ways in which caring expresses itself. Emphasis on the ontical category is particularly important as we challenge the tendency to reduce caring to its feeling, emotive expression. I have characterized these entities of caring as the five C's, compassion, competence, confidence, conscience, and commitment (1984, 1987).

The five C's are not mutually exclusive, but they provide a way to identify and name specific expressions of caring. Because of time constraints, only a brief overview is possible in this paper.

Compassion is a way of living born out of an awareness of our relationships to all living creatures. It is a quality of presence which allows us to share with and make room for the other. Compassion asks us to go,

> . . . where it hurts, to enter into the places of pain, to share the brokenness, fear, confusion, and anguish. Compassion challenges us to cry out with those in misery, to mourn with those who suffer loneliness, to weep with those in tears. Compassion requires us to be weak with the weak, vulnerable with the vulnerable, and powerless with the powerless. Compassion means full immersion in the condition of being human [McNeill, Morrison, Nouwen, 1982, p. 4].

Compassion gives to the cold, scientific world of technology an infusion of the spirit (Hellegers, 1975, p. 113).

Competence is the state of having the knowledge, judgment, skills, energy, experience, and motivation required to respond appropriately to the demands of our profession. There is a mutual relationship between compassion and competence; one presupposes the other. Competence without compassion can be brutal and inhuman. Compassion without competence can be a meaningless, if not harmful, intrusion into the life of a person needing care. Competence divorced from care is characterized by a dominance over the other that depersonalizes. It represents a mis-use of power symbolized by the up-the-ladder syndrome, a competitive, hierarchical mentality (Fox, 1979).

We all know how destructive the competitive mentality in nursing is, how destructive it is to community life, and the extent to which it suffocates the very source of caring energy. We experience the conflicts of power-seeking and competition within our professional relationships, and perhaps merit the observation that, when we deny our call to servanthood, to care, "compassion becomes spiritual stardom," compassion turned competition (McNeill, Morrison, Nouwen, 1982, p. 38).

Caring, as the human mode of being, as our way of being in the world with others, is expressed in a truly authentic way when we aim for excellence in whatever roles we find ourselves engaged, as educators, practitioners, researchers, or managers. Caring demands competence of the highest order. It is uncontaminated power, a power that calls the other to freedom.

Confidence is a term that subsumes all that fosters trusting relationships. Caring fosters trust without dependency; communicates truth without violence; and creates a relationship of respect without paternalism or maternalism, and without engendering a response born of fear or powerlessness. It enables freedom, creating spaces in our lives where we and others are free to be ourselves.

Conscience refers to a sensitive, informed sense of the moral fitness of things; a compass directing our behavior. Conscience is the caring person attuned to the moral nature of things. Conscience is the "call of care and manifests itself as care" (Heidegger, 1962, p. 319).

While caring as the human mode of being is not an ethical imperative, caring responds to ethical imperatives. Professional caring is reflected in a moral awareness that is fine-tuned by the discipline of knowledge and moral inquiry that forms a mature conscience.

Commitment is a complex personal response characterized by the convergence between our desires and our obligations, and by a deliberate choice to act in accordance with them. In Mayeroff's philosophical analysis of caring (1971), commitment subsumes the quality of devotion. According to his analysis, in devotion there is a convergence between what I want to do, and what I ought to do. Devotion (commitment) is essential to caring.

Commitment, then, is a quality of investment of self in a task, a person, a choice or career; a quality so internalized as a value that what I am obligated to do is not regarded as a burden. Rather, it is a call which draws me to a conscious, willing, and positive response.

The five C's present a broad framework for categories of human response within which professional caring is expressed. Specific manifestations of caring are actualized in compassionate and competent acts; in relationships qualified by trust; through informed, sensitive moral inquiry and decision making; and through commitment and fidelity to the choices we have made. I suggest educators, practitioners, researchers, and managers can be challenged to identify relevant, specific themes in stories and dialogue that document the evidence of these themes in the daily lives of caring professionals.

CONCLUSION

As I reviewed the nursing literature in preparation for this conference, I could not help perceive the consistency between the ideas of the curriculum revolution and those of a great educator, John Henry Cardinal Newman (1801–1890). In a well-known Western classic, *The Idea of a University,* (1959), Newman talks about knowledge viewed in relation to professional skill. His concept of intellect and intellectual development is anything but a slavish fixation on specific, mechanical behaviors or predetermined behavioral responses. In speaking of the nature of intellectual development, Newman refers to "an acquired faculty of judgment, of clear-sightedness, of sagacity, of wisdom, of philosophical reach of mind, and of intellectual self-possession and repose" (p. 171). Newman's reflections are relevant because, while we unveil the fallacies and the violence of some contemporary educational practices, we ought not be, and I hope we are not, anti-intellectual.

This trap of anti-intellectualism is extremely important to avoid because it is capable of spelling the downfall of our determination to preserve the centrality of caring in nursing. As my brief excursion through an ontology of caring and through some of its ontical expressions is intended to demonstrate, caring, as our human mode of being in the world, involves a total human response. In my introduction, I tried to capture some of the themes of our programs and in recent nursing literature. It is important to note that our stand is counterculture. For the values expressed in the curriculum revolution and for the goals to which we aspire in reclaiming the primacy of caring in nursing, the culture in which we live is, for the most part, functionless. Perhaps to some nurses, this is a shattering revelation.

This conference has brought us together in this wonderful, life-giving place to take up the challenge of our "extraordinary opportunity to address the many pressing ills of our current system" (Hawken, 1990, p. B). The ills of our system are within our own ranks, as well as constitutive of the way health care services are organized and administered. The ills come from a society in which we live and have shaped, and from a culture predominately fixated on the sensate. Many forces from within our profession as well as from society at large militate against our primary, human call to care. As a profession, we need a greater consciousness of this reality. We can take heart in our capacity and great potential to transform the system and the world around us. Nouwen puts it well when he reminds his readers,

> Every human being has a great, yet often unknown, gift to care, to be compassionate, to become present to the other, to listen, to hear and to receive. If that gift would be set free and made available, miracles would take place. [1974, p. 70]

We must move beyond the sensate to recapture the transcendent values which are the soul of nursing; and to reclaim as part of our universe of reflection, study, and research, the metaphysical and spiritual domains of knowledge and experience. The crisis we experience is not a bad phenomenon. As we struggle between the "no-longer and the not-yet" (Rowe, 1980) this crisis is our reminder that there is a vacuum that needs to be filled. There are alternatives.

I close these reflections with an ancient Roman myth which reminds us that our truest name is "care." When we cease to care, we cease to be human. Our humanity is the ground for our professional identity.

> Once when 'Care' was crossing a river, she saw some clay; she thoughtfully took up a piece and began to shape it. While she was meditating on what she had made, Jupiter came by. 'Care' asked him to give it spirit, and this he gladly granted. But when she wanted her name to be bestowed upon it, he forbade this, and demanded that it be given his name instead. While 'Care' and Jupiter were disputing, Earth arose and desired that her own name be conferred on the creature, since she had furnished it with part of her body. They asked Saturn to be their arbiter, and he made the following decision, which seemed a just one: "Since you, Jupiter, have given its spirit, you shall receive that spirit at its death; and since you, Earth, have given its body, you shall receive its body. But since 'Care' first shaped this creature, she shall possess it as long as it lives. And because there is now a dispute among you as to its name, let it be called 'homo,' for it is made out of humus (earth)." [Heidegger, 1962/1969]

BIBLIOGRAPHY

Allen, D. G. (1990). The curriculum revolution: Radical revisioning of nursing education. *Journal of Nursing Education, 29,* 312–316.

Bellah, R. N., Madsen, R., Sullivan, W., Swidler, A., & Tipton, S. (1985). *Habits of the heart.* New York: Harper & Row.

Bevis, E. O., & Murray, J. P. (1990). The essence of the curriculum revolution: Emancipatory teaching. *Journal of Nursing Education, 29,* 326–331.

Burrell, D., & Hauerwas, S. (1974). Speer's inside the Third Reich: Self-deception and autobiography: Theological and ethical reflections on. *Journal of Religious Ethics, 2,* 99–117.

Chinn, P. L. (1990). GOSSIP: A transformative art for nursing education. *Journal of Nursing Education, 29,* 318–321.

Cooperative Institutional Research Program. (1985). *New report tracks 20-year shift in freshmen attitudes, values and life goals.* Newsletter, American Council on Education. Los Angeles: University of California.

de Tocqueville, A. (1969). *Democracy in America.* (G. Lawrence, Trans.). New York: Doubleday.

de Tornyay, R. (1990). The curriculum revolution. *Journal of Nursing Education, 29,* 292–294.

Diekelmann, N. (1990). Nursing education: Caring, dialogue, and practice. *Journal of Nursing Education, 23,* 300-305.

Dubay, T. (1973). *Caring: A biblical theology of community.* Denville, NJ: Dimension Books.

Fox, M. (1979). *A spirituality named compassion.* Minneapolis: Winston Press.

Gaylin, W. (1979). *Caring.* New York: Alfred A. Knopf, Avon Books.

Hawken, P. (1990, December). *Letter.* In NLN program, "Curriculum Revolution: Community Building and Activism." New York: National League for Nursing.

Heidegger, M. (1962/1969). *Being and time.* (J. Macquarrie & E. Robinson, Trans.). London: SCM Press; New York: Harper & Row.

Hellegers, A. (1975). Compassion with competence. *America, 133,* 113–116.

Kelsey, M. (1981). *Caring.* New York: Paulist Press.

May, R. (1969). *Love and will.* New York: W. W. Norton & Co.

Mayeroff, M. (1971). *On caring.* New York: Harper & Row, Perennial Library.

Moccia, P. (1990). No sire, it's a revolution. *Journal of Nursing Education, 29,* 307–311.

McNeill, D. P., Morrison, D. A., & Nouwen, H. J. M. (1982). *Compassion: A reflection on the Christian life.* New York: Darton, Longman & Todd.

Newman, J. H. C. (1959). *The idea of a university.* Doubleday & Co., Inc.; Image Books.

Nouwen, H. J. M. (1974). *Out of solitude.* Notre Dame, IN: Ave Maria Press.

Roach, M. S. (1984). *Caring: The human mode of being, implications for nursing.* Toronto: University of Toronto.

Roach, M. S. (1987). *The human act of caring: A blueprint for the health professions.* Ottawa: Canadian Hospital Association.

Roach, M. S. (In press). *The call to consciousness: Compassion in today's health world.* Paper presented at the 12th Annual Caring Conference, International Association for Human Caring, University of Texas Health Science Center, Houston, TX.

Rowe, S. C. (1980). *Living beyond crisis: Essays on discovery and being in the world.* New York: Pilgrim Press.

Solzhenitsyn, A. (1978). *A world split apart.* New York: Harper & Row.

Sorokin, P. A. (1942). *The crisis of our age.* New York: E. P. Dutton.

Sorokin, P. A. (1964). *The basic trends of our times.* New Haven, CT: College and University Press.

Speer, A. (1971). *Inside the Third Reich.* (R. Winston & C. Winston, Trans.). New York: Macmillan Co.; Avon Publishers.

Tanner, C. A. (1990). Reflections on the curriculum revolution. *Journal of Nursing Education, 29,* 295–299.

Waters, V. (1990). Associate degree nursing and curriculum revolution II. *Journal of Nursing Education, 29,* 322–325.